HEIDELBERG SCIENCE LIBRARY | Volume 4

Biology of Antibiotics

Hans Zähner and

Werner K. Maas

Springer-Verlag

New York · Heidelberg · Berlin | 1972

Professor Hans Zähner
Director
Institut für Mikrobiologie
der Universität Tübingen
West Germany

Werner K. Maas
Professor of Microbiology
New York University School of Medicine
New York, New York

© 1972 by Springer-Verlag New York Inc.
Softcover reprint of the hardcover 1st edition 1972

Library of Congress Catalog Card Number 76-164963.

ISBN-13: 978-0-387-90034-6   e-ISBN-13: 978-1-4613-9373-3
DOI: 10.1007/978-1-4613-9373-3

Preface

This book is based on Hans Zähner's Biologie der Antibiotica, published in 1965.

There is a vast literature on antibiotics, covering chemical, pharmacological, and clinical aspects. We have made no attempt to cover this literature comprehensively. Our effort is directed toward discussing antibiotics as biological agents. They are substances produced by living cells, yet they are able to inhibit the growth of living cells — in many cases even the cells that produce them. We have taken this apparent biological paradox as our point of departure and have tried to look in this light at the production of antibiotics and at their mode of action. In a sense antibiotics are comparable to mutations. They are useful as tools in the study of metabolism by blocking specific reactions. At the same time their mode of origin and their effects on the organisms that produce them are interesting problems in their own right. We have tried to incorporate both aspects into our considerations.

This little book, designed for biology students and medical students, provides them with a framework into which to fit more specialized and detailed information on antibiotics. We have tried to present an overall picture of the actions of antibiotics on sensitive organisms and of the problems that arise during their use (for example, drug resistance) and at the same time to sketch out the biological background against which to consider the actions of antibiotics, such as the sources of antibiotics in nature and their biosyntheses in relation to the metabolism of the organisms that produce them.

Tübingen, November 25, 1970   Hans Zähner
                                                     Werner K. Maas

Contents

Contents

Chapter 1

Introduction

What are antibiotics? Why are they formed in nature? These two questions are discussed in this introductory chapter.

Antibiotics can be defined as substances produced by living organisms, which in low concentrations are able to inhibit growth of other organisms. This is a formal definition, and by and large it is valid. As with most definitions though, there are exceptions. For example, enzymes that are excreted by microorganisms and that by catalyzing the breakdown of proteins or carbohydrates inhibit the growth of other microbes are not considered to be antibiotics.

Over the years, as more and more antibiotics have been discovered, it has been found that most of them, especially those of medical importance, fall into the general category of *secondary metabolites*. Perhaps the simplest way to acquire an impression of these substances is to observe their formation. Among microorganisms their taxonomic distribution is restricted, and among bacteria we find them to be produced largely by certain spore-forming groups (Bacilli and Actinomycetes). During its normal life cycle such an organism will grow in an appropriate culture medium until it has produced the maximum number of cells it is capable of forming under the particular conditions. The limitation may be set by the supply of oxygen, by the amount of the carbon and energy source supplied, or by other nutritional or environmental factors. Once the culture has stopped growing, it enters the stationary phase, followed eventually by death or alternatively by spore formation. More is said about the growth of bacteria in Chapter 3. Usually at this stage — after the cells have stopped dividing — secondary metabolites begin to be produced. Their production continues for a certain length of time, which may be either longer or shorter than the active growth period of the culture, and it then ceases. Secondary metabolites are often produced in large

1

Table 1-1   Classes of Organic Compounds in Which Secondary Metabolites Are
Found

Amino sugars	Lactones	Pyrones
Anthocyanins	Macrolides	Pyrroles
Anthraquinones	Naphthalenes	Pyrrolines
Aziridines	Naphthoquinones	Pyrrolizines
Benzoquinones	Nucleosides	Quinolines
Coumarins	Oligopeptides	Quinolinols
Diazines	Phenazines	Quinones
Epoxides	Phenoxazinones	Salicylates
Ergoline alkaloids	Phthaldehydes	Terpenoids
Flavonoids	Piperazines	Tetracyclines
Glutaramides	Polyacetylenes	Tetronic acids
Glycosides	Polyenes	Triazines
Hydroxylamines	Pyrazines	Tropolones
Indole derivatives	Pyridines	

amounts, of the same order of magnitude as the dry weight of the
culture, and for the most part they are excreted into the culture
medium.

What is the chemical nature of secondary metabolites? They are
a diverse group of compounds, most of them of relatively low molecular weight. An awareness of this diversity may be gained from an
inspection of Table 1-1, which lists some of the classes of compounds
found among secondary metabolites, including classes that contain
antibiotics. It should be noted that, in spite of the large variety of
compounds, classes to which primary metabolites belong (amino acids,
sugars, and intermediates of carbohydrate metabolism, fatty acids,
and others) are largely absent. A characteristic feature of secondary
metabolism is that any given organism usually produces an array of
related compounds belonging to the same class. Another feature of
this type of metabolism is that a large number of substances arises
from relatively few intermediates of primary metabolism. These
aspects of secondary metabolism are discussed in Chapter 4.

In contrast to primary metabolites, secondary metabolites are not
essential for growth of the organism. Primary metabolites are either
building blocks for macromolecules, intermediates in reactions generating energy-rich compounds (ATP), or parts of coenzymes. Secondary metabolites have no such vital roles in metabolism. Yet it seems
likely that secondary metabolism does have a useful function in the

life of the organism, as shown in some cases (especially of sporulating bacteria), by inferior viability of mutant strains unable to carry out some steps in secondary metabolism. Presumably this type of metabolism protects the cell against environmental or internally generated hazards that arise during the resting phase. One usually thinks of microorganisms as living in a world in which all they do is grow and divide, but in nature as well as in artificial cultures, sooner or later the suspending medium becomes growth-limiting. It then becomes necessary for the organism to survive under such conditions until the environment changes and will again support its growth.

Secondary metabolism occurs also in fungi, higher plants, and to some extent in animals. Among the latter two, because of the intermingling between growing and differentiating cells, it is not so simple to draw a distinction, in terms of timing, between primary and secondary metabolism, as it is in microorganisms.

As we mentioned, most antibiotics are secondary metabolites, and what we have said about secondary metabolism applies to most of them. There are, however, a few antibiotics that are primary metabolites, being formed during the growth of the organism. The polypeptide antibiotic nisin is an example.

With the background of secondary metabolism presented here we can now ask the second question: Why do organisms produce antibiotics? They are growth-inhibitory substances, and moreover in many instances they inhibit the growth of the organisms that produce them. Before embarking on a further discussion, we admit that we do not know what their functions, if any, are, and what follows is therefore largely speculative.

Some of the possible roles that have been assigned to antibiotics are "useless" ones, such as waste products of cell metabolism or the breakdown products of macromolecules; or "useful" ones for the metabolism of the producing cell, such as food-storage, or useful ones for the life of the cell in its natural environment, such as inhibiting the growth of neighboring organisms. They have also been considered as biochemical vestiges that once had a useful function but have lost it. Without going into a detailed discussion of these possibilities we can say that probably none of these is correct, at least not as a primary function. We must remember that the purpose of secondary metabolism is to protect the cells against adverse conditions arising during the resting phase. Any function that may be assigned to antibiotics must be sought in this context.

A possible function of secondary metabolism is to prevent during the resting phase the accumulation of primary metabolites that may be harmful to the cell. Secondary metabolites, as we have mentioned, are formed from intermediates of primary metabolism. In that sense antibiotics and other secondary metabolites would be primarily the end products of "detoxification" enzymes, and their biological activity would be accidental, the important biological feature being the process of secondary metabolism per se.

It does not seem likely, however, that among all these biologically active substances, many of which can inhibit growth of the cells that produce them, some do not fulfill some sort of useful function. For example, it may be detrimental for a cell in a poor environment to try to synthesize macromolecules. Many antibiotics are inhibitors of macromolecular synthesis, and they may therefore be useful in preventing abortive attempts of cells to synthesize macromolecules.

As an extension of the idea that antibiotics participate in the control of macromolecular synthesis, we may consider the restricted distribution of these substances in nature. Among microorganisms, antibiotics are mainly found in species that have the ability to sporulate. It is possible, therefore, that the production of some antibiotics is related to the ability of an organism to sporulate. In bacilli, it has been demonstrated that the production of antibiotics occurs during the early stages of spore formation. It is likely that these antibiotics function as regulators of macromolecular synthesis. As sporulation may be considered as a process of differentiation, antibiotics active in this process are thus agents of differentiation.

These speculations lead us to define a central function of some antibiotics in the life of the organism that produces them. Admittedly there is no direct evidence for such a role of antibiotics, but then little is known (in contrast to primary metabolism) about the physiology of sporulation, although it has been studied extensively. A word of caution against generalizing about physiological roles of antibiotics: The production of antibiotics during secondary metabolism is extremely variable, the proportion among secondary metabolites produced being very much dependent on environmental conditions. This argues against all antibiotics being involved in vital processes, and emphasizes that in regard to biological functions we may be dealing with a very heterogeneous group.

In addition to a role in the metabolism of the organism that produces them, there is the possibility that in some cases the excretion of antibiotics has a selective advantage for the producer because of inhibition of growth of surrounding organisms. This is an incidental role that presumably has evolved secondarily and represents an "extra bonus" of the process of antibiotics production.

In summary, most antibiotics are produced during the resting phase of microbial growth, as a result of a type of metabolism, called secondary metabolism, which is different from that occurring during growth and division and is concerned with maintaining the cell during this phase of its life. This fact, together with the restricted taxonomic distribution of antibiotics, mainly among sporulating organisms, has invited speculation as to a possible role of some antibiotics in protecting the organism during the resting phase and, in some cases, in setting up or maintaining a differentiated state prerequisite to spore formation. There is not direct evidence for such a role of antibiotics, and such functions are suggested mainly on the basis of their being biologically active compounds. The alternative would be that the biological activity of these compounds is fortuitous and of no significance in secondary metabolism. The great variability observed in the production of secondary metabolites calls for a cautious attitude in assigning functions to antibiotics in resting-phase metabolism.

In the pages to follow we first discuss the taxonomic distribution of antibiotic-producing organisms (Chapter 2), then some general methods used in the study of antibiotics, together with the principles underlying these methods (Chapter 3). After this we deal with the biosynthesis (Chapter 4) and the mode of action (Chapter 5) of antibiotics, together with resistance developed to their actions (Chapter 6). Finally (Chapter 7) we deal with possible future studies on antibiotics.

We would like to emphasize again that the theme of this book is "biology of antibiotics," that is, not only a consideration of their uses by man but also a general treatment of their role in nature. However, a large part of this book is concerned with aspects relevant to medicine and other human endeavors. In addition we have purposely chosen as illustrative examples those antibiotics that are clinically useful.

References

WEINBERG, E. G., "Biosynthesis of Secondary Metabolites: Role of Trace Metals," in *Advances in Microbial Physiology*, Vol. 4., A. H. Rose and J. F. Wilkinson, eds., Academic Press, Inc. London and New York, 1970.

WOODRUFF, H. B., "The Physiology of Antibiotic Production: The Role of the Producing Organism," in *Biochemical Studies of Antimicrobial Drugs*, B. A. Newton and P. E. Reynolds, eds., Cambridge University Press, London, 1966.

Chapter 2

The Taxonomic Distribution of Antibiotic-
Producing Organisms

We shall make a few comments on limitations imposed on the detection of antibiotics before discussing the distribution of antibiotic-producers among living organisms.

1. With the commonly used procedures it is not possible to test all types of microorganisms for the production of antibiotics. For example, obligatory parasites are excluded, not because they lack biosynthetic capabilities, but because we have no way of determining antibiotics they may produce.

2. Each group of investigators engaged in the search for new antibiotics usually concentrates its efforts on a limited number of organisms. This has tended to produce a biased selection of organisms, in spite of the availability of generally applicable testing methods.

3. The conditions of testing impose limitations on the detection of antibiotics because of the limited number of indicator strains that can be used, the time of exposure of these strains to the potential antibiotic-producing strains, and the chosen culture conditions in general. Negative evidence for antibiotics-production in this case, therefore, is of much less value than is positive evidence.

4. In the literature on the distribution of antibiotics one often encounters data that were collected for other purposes and in which descriptions of antibiotic activity are fragmentary. For constructing a complete survey of antibiotic-producers it is desirable to have data from as wide a source as possible, but to be reliable, they have to contain a thorough description of an antibiotic, including chemical characterization.

Taking all these limitations into account, it still remains a fact that the taxonomic distribution of antibiotic-producing organisms is

Table 2-1   Distribution of Antibiotic-Producing Organisms

Producing organism	Number	Percent of total number of described producers
Pseudomonadales	11	1.2
Eubacteriales	70	7.7
	(53 are *Bacilli*)	—
Actinomycetales	529	58.2
Fungi	165	18.1
Algae and lichens	8	0.9
Higher plants	1·10	12.1
Animals	16	1.8
	909	100

(compiled from Korzybski *et al.* 1967)

very much restricted. This is shown in Table 2-1, which lists the distribution of organisms producing well-characterized antibiotics. (The data were compiled in 1967.) If we take all published descriptions of antibiotics into account, the total number of antibiotics would be greater, but it would hardly change the distribution.

Figure 2-1 shows a phylogenetic scheme for the fungi. Chemotherapeutically useful antibiotics have been found only among members of the order *Aspergillales*. Figure 2-1 shows some of the important antibiotics and the species that produce them. A few other groups of fungi also produce antibiotics, though not clinically useful ones. For example, polyacetylenes are produced by certain *Basidiomycetes;* certain *fungi imperfecti,* especially *Fusarium* species, produce enniatins, enniatin-like compounds, and quinone antibiotics. Compared to *Aspergillales* the number of other antibiotic-producers is small.

Bacterial taxonomy is at a much less advanced stage than taxonomy of the fungi, and it is futile to attempt the construction of a phylogenetic scheme comparable to that in Fig. 2-1. A scheme of this kind prepared by Hütter for a single group, the *Actinomycetales,* is shown in Fig 2-2. Again producers of medically and otherwise important antibiotics are indicated, and here they are found mainly among the genera *Streptomyces* and *Nocardia.* These two genera are closely related and belong to the same family. Thus among actinomycetes, as among fungi, only one group of closely related genera produces clinically important antibiotics. What is striking among the antibiotics

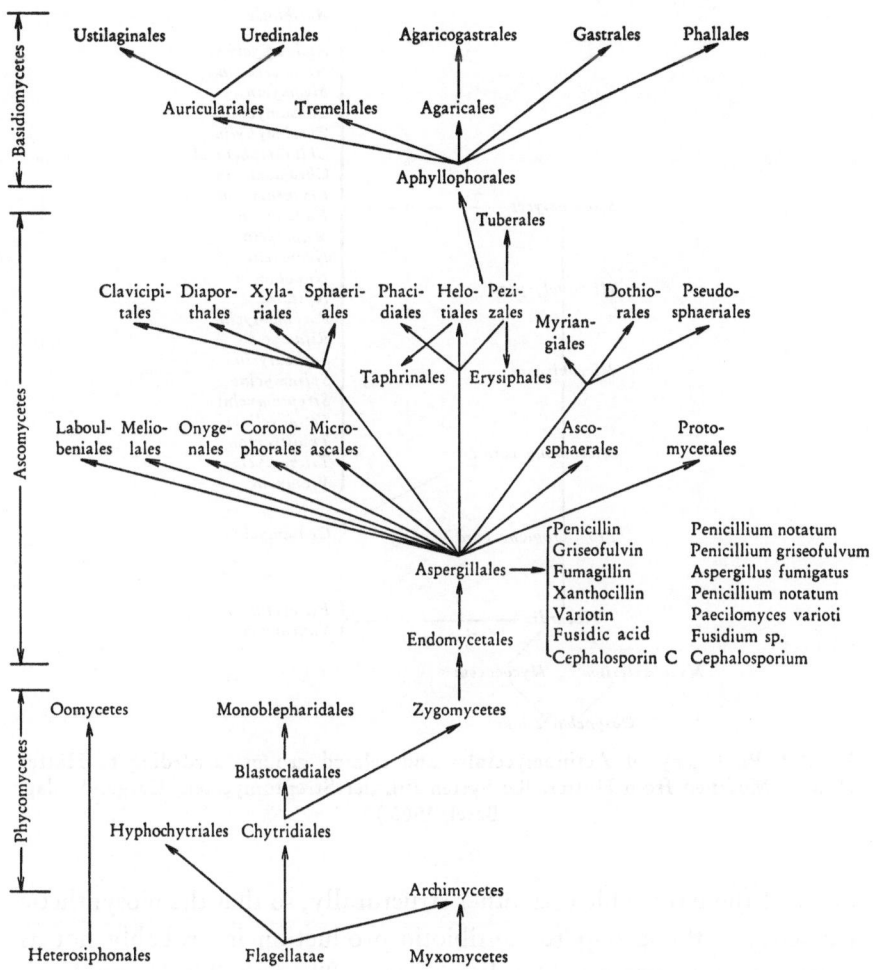

Fig. 2-1. Phylogeny of fungi, according to Gäumann (1964). Chemotherapeutically useful antibiotics, produced by *Aspergillales,* are indicated.

produced by actinomycetes is the great variety of substances, both in regard to chemical structure and mode of action. Actinomycetes have contributed a number of new classes to the catalogue of natural products, such as the macrolides, sideromycins, macrotetrolides, anthracyclines, and others.

Figure 2-3 shows a classification scheme of the *Eubacteriales* according to Bergey. Antibiotics are produced only by the *Bacillaceae.* Five important antibiotics are indicated, all of which are polypeptides.

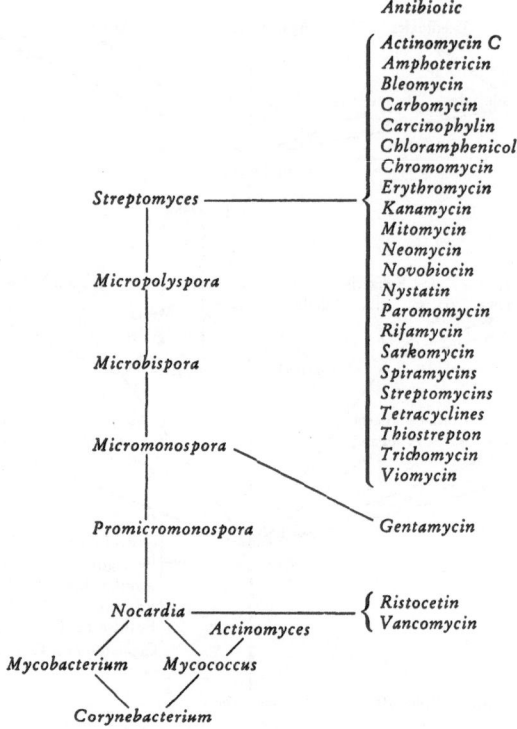

Fig. 2-2. Phylogeny of Actinomycetales and related groups, according to Hütter (1966). (Modified from Hütter, R.; Systematik der Streptomyceten, Karger-Verlag, Basel, 1966.)

Some of these resemble each other structurally, so that the biosynthetic capacity of this group for antibiotic production is probably not as great as may be suggested by their number. These antibiotics are, however, very different from each other in their mode of action. It may be mentioned that polymyxin and colistin are very active against gram-negative bacteria and only weakly active against gram-positive bacteria, which is an unusual situation among antibiotics. Gramicidin S, bacitracin, and tyrothricin, like most other antibiotics, are more active against gram-positive bacteria.

It can be seen from Figs. 2-1, 2-2, and 2-3 that the production of a given antibiotic is usually confined to a single group of closely related organisms. This "rule of specificity" holds for all therapeutically important antibiotics. If we consider other well-characterized antibiotics, the rule still holds for several hundred more. Exceptions to this rule

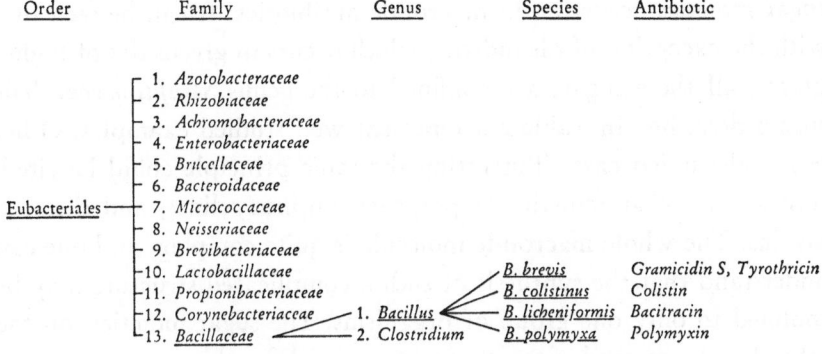

Order	Family	Genus	Species	Antibiotic

Fig. 2-3. Antibiotic-producers among *Eubacteriales*.

Table 2-2   Exceptions to the "Rule of Specificity"

Antibiotic	Producing organism
Cephalosporin N	*Cephalosporium* (Fungi Imperfecti *Streptomyces*
Citrinin	Leaves of *Crotalaria crispata* *Penicillium* *Streptomyces*
Fusidic acid (Ramycin)	*Fusidium* (Fungi Imperfecti, belongs probably to the ascomycetes) *Cephalosporium* *Mucor ramannianus* (a phycomycete)
Beta-nitropropionic acid (Bovino- cidin)	*Streptomyces* *Aspergillus* Constituent of a glycoside in higher plants
Various phenazines	*Streptomyces* *Pseudomonas iodinum*
9-(B-D-riboturanosyl)-purine (Nebularin)	*Agaricus nebularis* (a basidiomycete)

are listed in Table 2-2. The "rule of specificity" applies not only to single substances but also to whole classes of substances and to building blocks of antibiotics, such as sugar moieties. Thus in regard to classes of compounds, macrolide and polyene antibiotics have been demonstrated only in cultures of actinomycetes. There they occur with high frequency, polyenes being found among 75 percent of freshly isolated strains, macrolides among 1 to 3 percent. Another group, the polyacetylene antibiotics, have so far been found only among basidiomycetes. In regard to specific moieties, Table 2-3 lists some of the sugar moieties occurring in macrolide antibiotics. It can be seen that with the exception of oleandrose, which occurs in glycosides of higher plants, all these sugars are confined to the genus *Streptomyces*. The sugars described in Table 2-3 represent well-studied examples. Other less well-studied cases illustrating the same principle could be cited, such as the sugar moieties of polyenes, anthracyclines, and chromomycins. The whole macrolide molecule is quite complex, and one can understand that the synthesis of such a complicated structure may be confined to only one group of organisms. The sugar moieties, on the other hand, are much simpler structures, and for this reason one may expect them to be distributed more widely. Yet the genetic capabilities for their production have been retained within only a very limited group of organisms. This is reminiscent of a group of dideoxy sugars that are confined in their occurrence mainly to certain enteric bacteria (Salmonella), where they form part of the surface O antigen.

In conclusion, in examining the distribution of antibiotic-producing species, we find it to be very restricted, mainly to certain microorganisms that are able to sporulate, and moreover, we find a great deal of specificity in regard to the kind of antibiotics produced by a given group of organisms. We have already indicated in Chapter 1 a possible explanation for the restricted evolution of antibiotics, namely that antibiotic production is part of the secondary metabolism characteristic of these sporulating organisms. The rule of specificity reflects further specializations among these groups. One final point can be made in regard to the restricted distribution: Considering that antibiotics are not absolutely essential for life and may be produced in copious amounts, organisms that evolved the capacity to produce them must be living in a relatively rich environment, with good supplies of nutrients. Conditions of plenty are not found too often, though they seem to be present in the soil in which antibiotic-producers are found.

References
Bacteria

BREED, R., E. MURRAY, and N. SMITH, *Bergey's Manual of Determinative Bacteriology*, 7th ed., The Williams & Wilkins, Baltimore, 1957.

HÜTTER, R., *Systematik der Streptomyceten*, Karger-Verlag, Basel, 1966.

JONES, D. and P. H. A. SNEATH: "Genetic Transfer and Bacterial Taxonomy", *Bacteriol. Rev.* 34, 40–81, 1970.

Table 2—3   Some Sugar Moieties of Macrolide Antibiotics

Sugar	Chemical structure	Component of	Formed by
Desosamine (picrosin)		Methymycin Picromycin Griseomycin Narbomycin Erythromycins Oleandomycin	Various species of *Streptomyces*
Mycaminose		Spiramycins Carbomycins Leucomycins Niddamycin Tylosin Acumycin Relomycin	Various species of *Streptomyces*
Torosamine		Spiramycins	*S. aureofaciens*
Angolosamine		Angolamycin	Various species of *Streptomyces*
Mycarose		Erythromycin Carbomycin Spiramycins Angolamycin Tylosin Leucomycin	Various species of *Streptomyces*
Oleandrose		Oleandomycin Cardiac glycosides	*S. antibioticus* Higher plants
Lankavose		Lankamycin Chalcomycin	Various species of *Streptomyces*

WAKSMAN, S. A., *The Actinomycetes*, Vol. 2, The Williams & Wilkins Company, Baltimore, 1960.

Fungi

GÄUMANN, E., *Die Pilze*, Birkhäuser-Verlag, Basel, 1964.
RAPER, K. B. and C. THOM, *A Manual of the Penicillia*, The Williams & Wilkins Company, Baltimore, 1949.
RAPER, K. B. and D. I. FENNELL, *The Genus Aspergillus*, The Williams & Wilkins Company, Baltimore, 1965.

Antibiotics

KORZYBSKI, T., Z. KOWSZYK-GINDIFER, and W. KURYLOWICZ, *Antibiotics, Origin, Nature and Properties*, Pergamon Press, Inc., New York, 1967.
MILLER, M. W., *The Pfizer Handbook of Microbial Metabolites*, McGraw-Hill, Inc., New York, 1961.
UMEZAWA, H., *Index of Antibiotics from Actinomycetes*, University of Tokyo Press, Tokyo; University Park Press, State College, Pa., 1967.
WAKSMAN, S. A., *The Actinomycetes*, Vol. 3, The Williams & Wilkins Company, Baltimore, 1962.

Chapter 3

Tests of Antibiotic Activity

In practical work, methods of testing are important either in the search for new antibiotics or for clinical sensitivity tests. The former requires testing of different organisms for the production of new antimicrobial agents and testing of natural products for antibiotic activity; the latter entails the testing of organisms isolated from patients for sensitivity to antibiotics used in therapy. In either type of work the choice of the method is conditioned by the biological problem to be investigated; however, as a general feature, for any work of this type it is important to distinguish between bacteristatic and bactericidal action of the antibiotic.

A bacteristatic agent inhibits growth without killing the organism; the bacteria resume normal growth after removal of the antibiotic. A bactericidal agent kills the organism. Exposure to the antibiotic is followed by a loss in viability that cannot be reversed when the antibiotic is removed. In practice this criterion is not always clear-cut. Some antibiotics may be either bacteristatic or bactericidal, depending on the experimental conditions employed. For example, at borderline concentrations an agent that is ordinarily bactericidal may become bacteristatic. As applied to microorganisms the concept of inhibition of growth ordinarily refers to populations rather than to individual organisms. Bacteristasis thus may result from an antibiotic killing some of the organisms while permitting growth of others, the end result being the maintenance of a constant number of viable organisms in a population.

The effectiveness of an antibiotic depends on a number of experimental variables, some of which we discuss now, before we discuss testing procedures. These variables are

1. the phase of growth and rate of growth of the organism;
2. the nature of the growth medium;

3. the concentration of the antibiotic;
4. the population density;
5. the rate at which resistant mutants arise.

In order to use testing methods rationally it is important to have an understanding of these factors and their relationship to the purpose for which the testing is being done.

Factors Affecting the Action of Antibiotics

Effect of Growth Phase and Growth Rate

Growth of bacteria can be measured easily and accurately, in terms of both mass and numbers. Effects on growth rate are therefore easily determined. Growth, however, is the end result of a large number of metabolic activities, and inhibition of growth does not tell us specifically which of these many activities has been altered. Nevertheless, growth can be varied in a controlled way, and we do know something about differences in metabolism under different conditions of growth. Studying the effect of an antibiotic under different conditions of growth may therefore yield useful information about the action of the drug on cell metabolism.

One of the simplest ways to study varying conditions of growth is to follow a bacterial culture during its normal growth cycle. This cycle is usually subdivided into different phases, which are depicted in Fig. 3-1.

a. Lag phase. This is a period of adjustment before the assumption of normal growth. There is an increase in bacterial mass, including

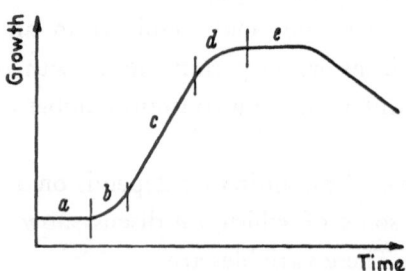

Fig. 3-1. Growth curve of a bacterial culture. For a description of phases, see the text.

proteins and nucleic acids, but no cell division and thus no increase in cell number.

b. This is a transitional period of accelerating growth.

c. Exponential (log) phase. Mass and cell number increase exponentially, with a constant generation time. During this phase the culture is in its most homogeneous state, with all the cells growing at the same rate and dividing at regular intervals.

d. This is a transitional period of decelerating growth, caused by exhaustion of an essential nutrient or an accumulation of a toxic factor.

e. Stationary phase. The limit of growth that can be supported under the particular conditions of culture has been reached. The number of viable bacteria remains constant at first; then after a variable length of time the bacteria begin to die at an exponential rate. Sporulation may occur here.

The division of the growth curve into these five phases is arbitrary. Also, the curve in Fig. 3-1 is schematic, and in actual experiments the lengths of the phases may be quite different from those shown in the figure. For example, the length of the lag phase depends on the physiological state of the inoculum. If the inoculum is taken from a culture in the exponential phase and is transferred into fresh medium of the same composition, there is no lag at all, and the culture enters the exponential phase immediately.

In terms of cell physiology we have some knowledge about each of these phases. For example, we know that during the lag phase protein and nucleic acid synthesis take place but cell division does not, and that during the stationary phase synthesis of many macromolecules has stopped but energy metabolism is continuing.

Let us now consider the effect of a given antibiotic on the various phases of growth of a culture. For an antibiotic to be effective it has to inhibit growth during the exponential phase. From exposure of a culture during stationary phase we can tell whether or not the substance kills nongrowing cells (in the case of bactericidal antibiotics) and whether or not it interferes with cellular respiration.

Exposure during the lag phase can be used to test for inhibition of synthesis of proteins and of nucleic acids. This kind of information, though crude, can be helpful in elucidating the mode of action of an antibiotic. For example, chloramphenicol, which is an inhibitor of protein synthesis, affects a culture during the lag phase and the exponential phase but not during the stationary phase.

There are other ways of varying the growth rate of a culture, such as limiting the supply of oxygen (anaerobic growth) or by growing a culture in a chemostat (a continuous culture device) with the supply of an essential metabolite limiting the growth rate. In regard to the former, much is known about the differences in metabolism between aerobic and anaerobic conditions, so that the testing of an antibiotic under these two kinds of conditions may provide valuable clues to the antibiotics' action on the cell. The chemostat permits the experimenter to set the growth rate by regulating the rate at which a limiting essential nutrient is supplied to the culture. It also permits him to maintain a culture in exponential growth for a prolonged period of time, since the medium is renewed continuously. Since with chemostat experiments any essential nutrient can be made growth-limiting, cell metabolism may be varied in a precise manner. For example, limiting the growth by limiting the nitrogen source, such as ammonia, will decrease the supply of building blocks for proteins and nucleic acids but presumably will have less effect on the generation of energy-rich bonds (ATP). Employment of these conditions should therefore accentuate the action of those antibiotics that inhibit growth by interfering with the formation of nitrogenous building blocks.

Effect of Medium Constituents

Since the nature of the growth medium can affect metabolism in many ways, it may affect sensitivity to antibiotics. For example, an antibiotic that acts by interfering with purine synthesis will inhibit the growth of an organism in a medium not containing purines but will have no effect when purines are supplied exogenously. The best-known example of reversal of inhibition by specific metabolites is the case of sulfonamides, which are antimetabolites but not antibiotics. Here the inhibition can be overcome either by a substrate (PAB) or by a product (folic acid) of the inhibited reaction. Among antibiotics this type of antagonism is found frequently, especially if one includes antibiotics that are not useful therapeutically. Some examples are shown in Table 3-1. These examples stress the importance of using chemically defined media wherever possible in order to detect antagonistic effects of medium constituents.

Besides these specific effects, the medium may affect sensitivity to antibiotics in nonspecific ways. For example, proteins present in the medium may bind the antibiotic and prevent its action. Attention must be given to this factor when media containing serum are used. The pH of the medium may influence the activity of the antibiotic, its stability, or its ability to be transported into the cell. Another factor is "general enrichment" of the medium that may determine the rate of growth and thus the population density at a given time. The relationship between growth rate and sensitivity to antibiotics has already been mentioned, and the role of the population density is discussed below.

Effect of Antibiotic Concentration

We have already mentioned that the same antibiotic may be bactericidal at one concentration and bacteristatic at lower concentrations. The effect of increasing the concentration of an antibiotic on the number of cellular reactions affected is discussed in Chapter 5.

Effect of Population Density

When an antibiotic acts as an antimetabolite by inhibiting activity of a specific enzyme within cells, no effect of population density on the effectiveness of the antibiotic would be expected since its concentration is usually in excess of that of enzyme molecules. This type of inhibition has been studied extensively with cell-free enzyme systems and can be described by Michaelis–Menten type of kinetics, in which the degree of inhibition is independent of the enzyme concentration. But with many antibiotics the action is a stoichiometric one, the antibiotic and the affected molecule being present in roughly the same concentrations under conditions of significant inhibition. Here the population density is important because it determines the concentration of the receptor sites for the antibiotic.

Figure 3-2 shows the effect of inoculum size on the activity of several agents that act in a stoichiometric fashion. In these experiments a serial dilution test was used to determine antibiotic activity (see below). In Fig. 3-3 *a* and *b* the same principle is illustrated, this time

Table 3-1 Some Antimetabolite Antibiotics and Their Metabolite Antagonists*

Antibiotic	Chemical structure	Formed by	Corresponding metabolite
Amino acid analogs			
Cycloserine	H_2C—CH—NH_2 (cyclic, $C{=}O$, N—H, O)	Various Streptomycetes	D-alanine
Hadacidin	$HC{=}O$ / N—OH / CH_2 / $COOH$	*Penicillium frequentans*	L-aspartic acid
DON 6-diazo-5-oxo-L-Norleucine	$HC{=}N{\equiv}N$ / $C{=}O$ / CH_2 / CH_2 / HC—NH_2 / $COOH$	Various Streptomycetes	L-glutamine
Azaserine	$HC{=}N{\equiv}N$ / $C{=}O$ / O / CH_2 / HC—NH_2 / $COOH$	Various Streptomycetes	L-glutamine

Analogs of vitamins

Bacimethrin   *Bacillus megatherium*   Thiamin

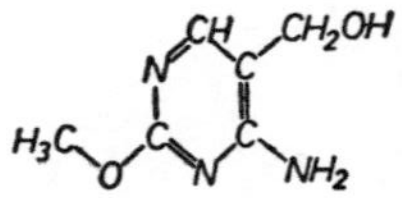

Analogs of sideramines

Ferrimycin A   Various Streptomycetes   Ferrioxamines (example: ferrioxamine B)

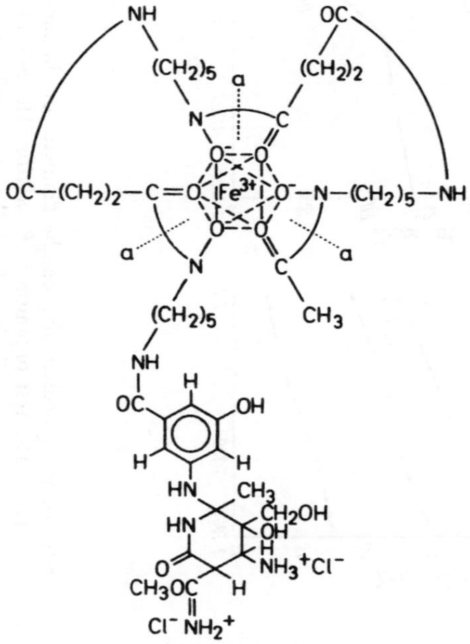

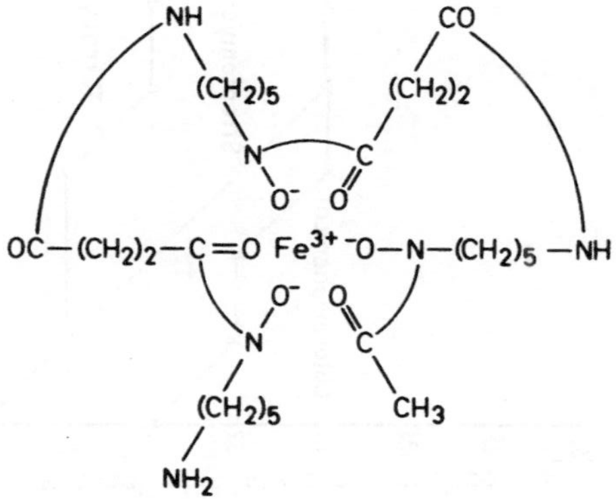

$C_{41}H_{87}O_{14}N_{10}Cl_2Fe$

* For purine and pyrimidine analogs see Figs. 4-1, 5-1, and 5-2.

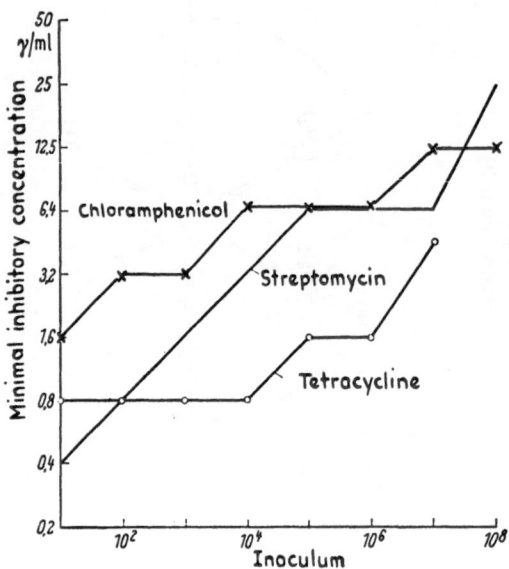

Fig. 3-2. Effect of the inoculum size on the minimal inhibitory concentration (MIC). The test organism is *E. coli*.

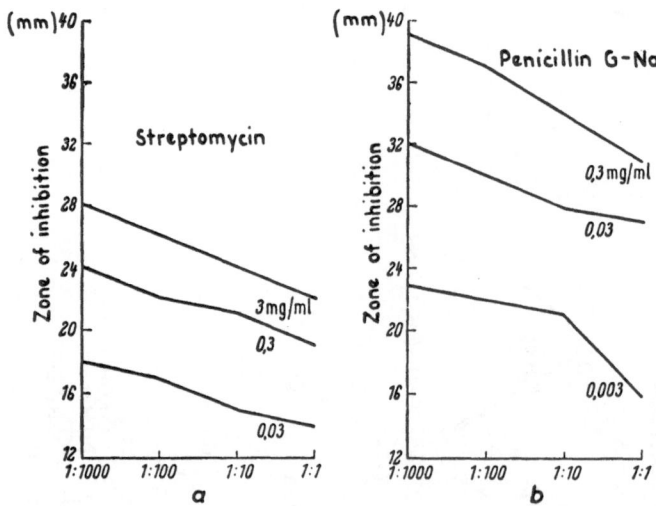

Fig. 3-3. Effect of the inoculum size on the diameter of the zone of inhibition in plate-diffusion tests. The test organism is *B. subtilis*. The inoculum size is given in terms of dilution of a fully grown culture.

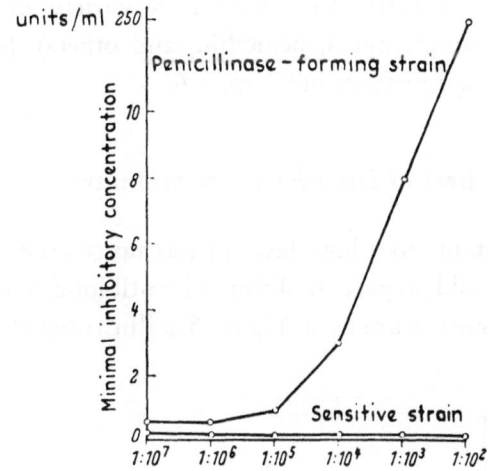

Fig. 3-4. Effect of inoculum size on MIC. The test organism: penicillinase-producing and penicillin-sensitive *S. aureus* strains.

using an agar-diffusion test. Note that in the latter method the diameter of the zone of inhibition is not directly proportional to the concentration of the antibiotic but rather to the logarithm of the concentration (Fig. 3-8). In this test, therefore, slight variations in diameter size represent large fluctuations in antibiotic concentration, and for this reason this method is prone to large experimental errors. This method is described in detail below.

The effect of inoculum size is apparent with organisms that produce and excrete an enzyme that destroys an antibiotic. For example, Fig. 3-4 shows a strain of *Staphylococcus aureus* which forms penicillinase. At low population densities the enzyme is not produced in sufficient amounts to prevent the killing action of penicillin, whereas at high population densities the rate of enzyme formation allows enough enzyme to be present to destroy the penicillin before it can kill the bacteria.

The genes for a number of different enzymes that inactivate some of the commonly used antibiotics are carried on extrachromosomal elements (plasmids), which are infectious and can be transmitted to bacteria belonging to the same or related species. For example, among enteric bacteria, such particles named R factors (resistance factors) enable the infected bacteria to inactivate a variety of antibiotics (chloramphenicol, streptomycin, penicillin, and others). More is said about infectious drug resistance in Chapter 6.

Effect of Drug-Resistant Mutants

If one-step mutants to a high level of resistance arise with a high frequency, one would expect abolition of antibiotic activity when sufficiently large inocula are used. Figure 3-5 illustrates this effect for

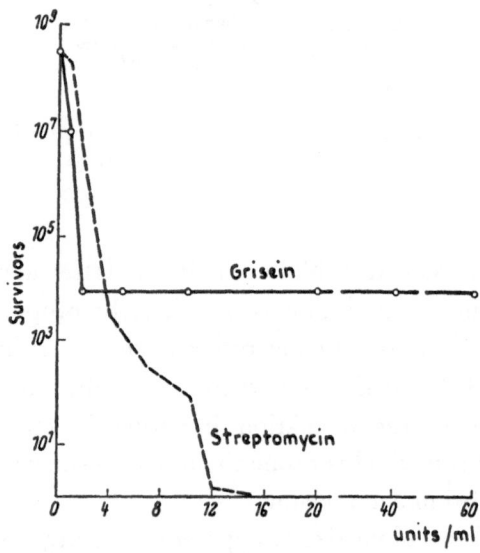

Fig. 3-5. Influence of concentration of grisein and streptomycin on the survival of *E. coli* on nutrient agar plates.

grisein and Fig. 3-6, for ferrimycin; a delay occurs in the outgrowth of the culture (Fig. 3-6) because only resistant mutants are able to grow. Figure 3-5 illustrates that about 1 per 100,000 bacteria in the culture survives, irrespective of the concentration of grisein used. One-step mutants to a high level of resistance can also arise with streptomycin, but here the frequency of resistant cells in a population is much lower than for grisein (Fig. 3-5).

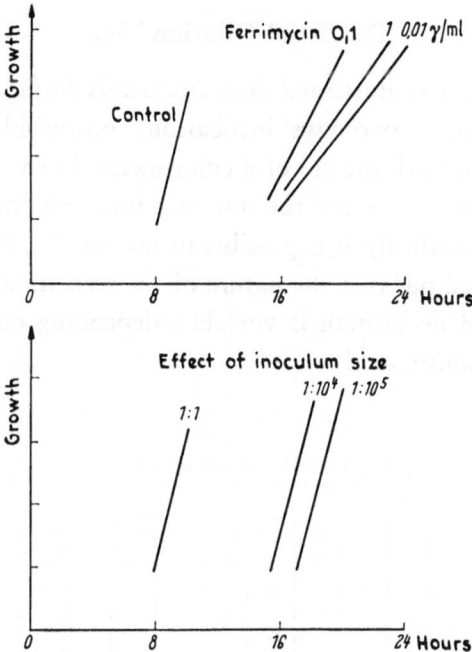

Fig. 3-6. Above: influence of different concentrations of ferrimycin on the out-growth of *B. subtilis*. Below: delay of outgrowth by the dilution of the inoculum, with constant concentration of ferrimycin.

Standard Methods

The techniques used for testing of antibiotic activity are technically simple and do not require elaborate apparatus. Difficulties may arise, however, in the reproducibility of the methods and, once these have been overcome, in the interpretation of the results. This is not surprising because we are using complex living organisms as indicator strains. It is important to keep this fact in mind, especially in regard to the variables discussed in the preceding section.

Three general tests are described that have proven to be of value in the routine assays of antibiotic activity. They are the serial-dilution test, the plate-diffusion test, and streaking on solid media containing different concentrations of the antibiotic. After that, a number of special testing methods are discussed. In all these tests it is the inhibition of growth that is being measured. Of particular importance is the determination of the antibiotic concentration that just inhibits growth, or minimal inhibiting concentration (MIC).

The Serial-Dilution Test

The procedure is illustrated diagramatically in Fig. 3-7. The tubes are read after one or two days' incubation, and turbidity is estimated either visually or with the aid of a colorimeter. For visual estimation, three-fold dilution steps are the minimal intervals that can be used, whereas photometrically it is possible to use smaller dilution steps. It should be pointed out that the nature of the transition range between full growth and no growth is variable, depending on the antibiotic and the test organism used.

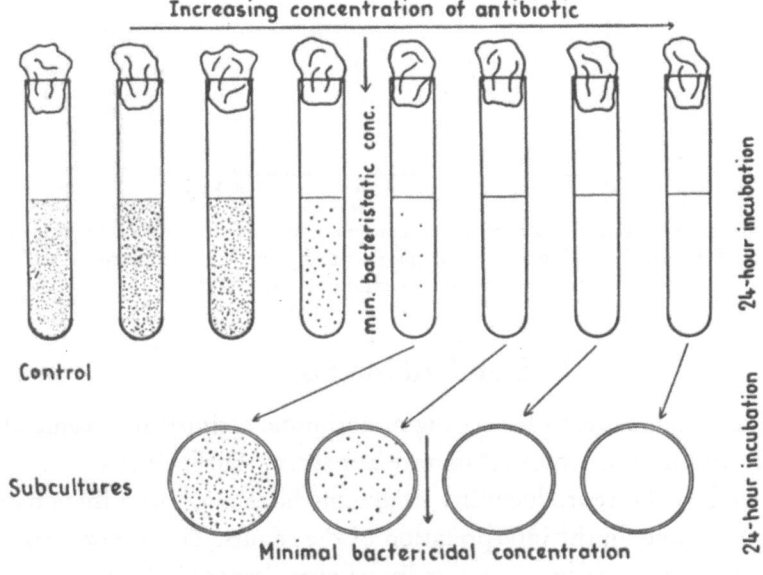

Fig. 3-7. The serial-dilution test.

Plate-Diffusion Tests

In these tests the organisms are seeded into the agar medium to give a fairly dense, uniform growth (10 to 100,000 bacteria per milliliter). The bacteria are added either directly to the melted agar medium at the time of pouring of the plates, or they are added in a second layer of "soft" agar on top of the agar medium. Either way may yield good results, the important point being uniform thickness

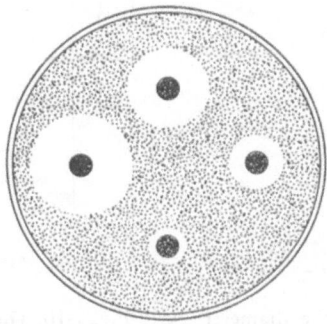

Fig. 3-8. The plate-diffusion test.

of the agar medium and the even distribution of the bacteria. The smaller the inoculum, the more sensitive the method, but the inoculum must be large enough to give a halo-type of growth with small colonies of uniform size (see Fig. 3-8). Once the plates are prepared, the substances to be tested are added. This may be done in several ways: the solution of the antibiotic may be pipetted into circular holes cut into the agar or it may be pipetted into cylinders consisting of glass, metal, or porcelain that have been set into the agar. Another, and probably the most widely used and exact, method is to apply filter paper disks to the surface of the agar that have been impregnated with a measured amount of the antibiotic. These disks are available commercially. After one to two days of incubation, the plates are read by measuring the diameter of the zone of inhibition (Fig. 3-8).

If standard conditions are adhered to, this test can be used quantitatively for the assay of antibiotic solutions of unknown concentrations. Under completely standardized conditions (inoculum size, composition and thickness of agar medium, incubation time, etc.) the diameter of the zone of inhibition is found to be proportional to the logarithm of the concentration of the antibiotic. This is illustrated for penicillin and *Bacillus subtilis* in Figs. 3-9 and 3-10. It is important to run each assay several times because small differences in the diameter of the zone of inhibition may represent large differences in antibiotic concentration. The concentration of the antibiotics in an unknown solution can most easily be measured by the comparison with a standard curve with known amounts of the antibiotic. Although this

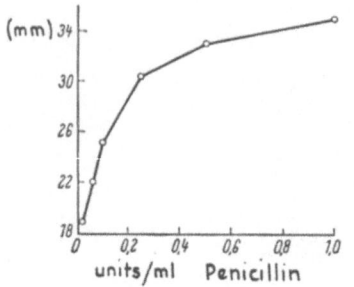

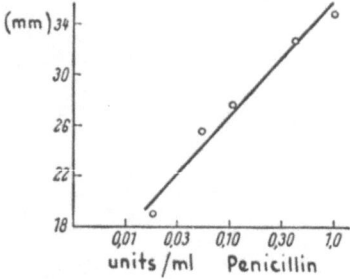

Fig. 3-9. Dependence of the diameter of the zone of inhibition on the concentration of the antibiotic. An example is effect of penicillin on the growth of B. subtilis.

Fig. 3-10. These are the same data as in Fig. 3-9, but the concentration of the antibiotic is plotted on a logarithmic scale.

method can be used with accuracy, its main utility is in the clinical laboratory for carrying out sensitivity tests, because for these tests precise quantitation is not required.

Serial Dilution Test on Solid Media

This method is advantageous in that several different organisms can be tested on the same plate. A series of agar plates is prepared containing ten-fold serial dilutions of the antibiotic to be tested and a control plate containing no antibiotic. The strains to be tested are then streaked on these plates, as shown in Fig. 3-11. The plates are examined after one day's incubation. Growth in the presence of the antibiotic is compared to that on the control plate. Figure 3-11 shows such a test with erythromycin and seven species of microorganisms.

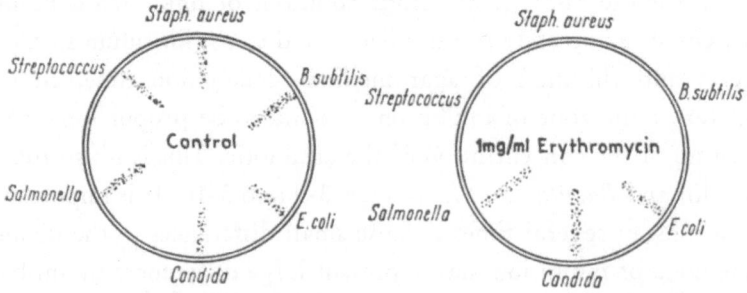

Fig. 3-11. Serial-dilution test on solid media. At left is the control without added antibiotic.

Table 3-2   Advantages and Disadvantages of Tests for Antibiotic Activity

Property	Test		
	1 *	2 +	3 §
Absolute concentration required for minimal inhibition can be determined	+	−	+
Test is very sensitive and accurate	+	−	−
Test requires relatively little work	−	+	+
Quantitative evaluation easily achieved with ± 10 percent accuracy	−	+	−
Information about a variety of organisms easily obtainable	−	−	+
Little danger of contamination	−	+	+
Can be adapted easily to distinguish between bacteristatic and bactericidal action	+	−	−

* serial dilution test — liquid medium
+ plate diffusion test
§ serial dilution test — solid medium

In Table 3-2 the advantages and disadvantages of the three test methods summarized.

Special Testing Methods

Now a few special procedures designed to answer certain specific questions are described. They illustrate how one can utilize microorganisms to answer very complicated questions in a simple manner. Here again it is necessary to keep in mind the limitations imposed by the experimental conditions.

A "Cross-Streak" Test

This method has been designed to screen actinomycetes for the production of antibiotics. It permits the testing of a large number of strains on one plate. First the potential antibiotic-producing actinomycete is streaked across a plate that is then incubated for 3 to 10 days at a temperature optimal for actinomycetes. After the streak has grown out, the indicator strains are streaked at right angles to it and the plate is again incubated, this time at the temperature for their optimal growth. As many as 10 strains can be tested on one plate.

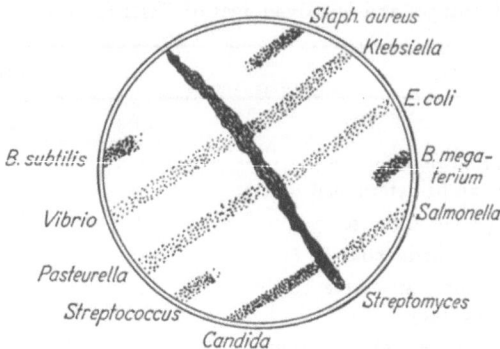

Fig. 3-12. Cross-streak test.

After the second incubation, the plate is examined. Antibiotic production is indicated by inhibition of growth of the indicator strains adjacent to the streak of the actinomycete. Figure 3-12 illustrates this method with a strain of *Streptomyces erythraeus,* which produces erythromycin.

This method is very simple and yields clear results. Although it has many advantages, such as the screening of large numbers of indicator strains and little danger of contamination, it has not been used widely in recent years. The reason is that most antibiotics that can be found with this method have already been found; new ones are rare. Furthermore, certain limitations make the application of this test difficult, for example, providing a good nutrient medium that will promote growth of the actinomycete as well as all the indicator strains.

The Antagonism Test

This method is suitable for testing substances suspected of antagonizing the action of an antibiotic. It is simple to execute, whereas the use of the other methods for this purpose, such as the serial-dilution test or agar-diffusion test is cumbersome and time-consuming. Two filter paper strips are placed on an agar plate across each other, the agar medium having been seeded with the test organism in the same manner as in the agar-diffusion test (Fig. 3-13). One of the strips is soaked in a solution of the antibiotic, the other in a solution of the suspected antagonist. In a case of competitive reversal of the inhibi-

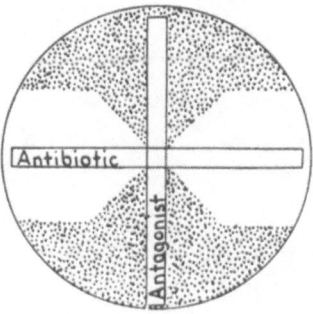

Fig. 3-13. Antagonism test. The inhibitor is ferrimycin; the antagonist is ferriox-amine B. The test organism is *B. subtilis*

tion the pattern shown in Fig. 3-13 is obtained after incubation of the plate. The diagonal borderlines represent the geometric locus of a constant inhibitor: antagonist ratio that just permits (or does not permit) growth. The test can be used for quantitative evaluations in a way similar to the simple agar-diffusion test.

Because this test is relatively insensitive it is not suitable for the detection of potentiation or synergism, in contrast to the test to be described next. The reason is that such effects are usually quite small, a stimulation by a factor of 3 to 10 of antibiotic activity being considered unusually high. Such increases are hardly detectable with certainty by this method because of logarithmic relationship between the zone of inhibition and the antibiotic concentration (Fig. 3-10), as already explained for the agar-diffusion test.

A Paper-Strip-Gradient Test

This test is suitable for detecting potentiating effects of substances that by themselves produce no effect. It is carried out as follows: First, a pour plate is prepared containing a gradient of antibiotic concentrations. This is achieved by pouring out the agar containing no antibiotic and letting it harden while the plate is in a slanted position. Then agar medium containing antibiotic is added, and the plate is now kept in a horizontal position. The gradient is established because of the overlapping slanted agar layers (see Fig. 3-14 *a*). The concentration of the antibiotic is chosen such that growth is inhibited to about

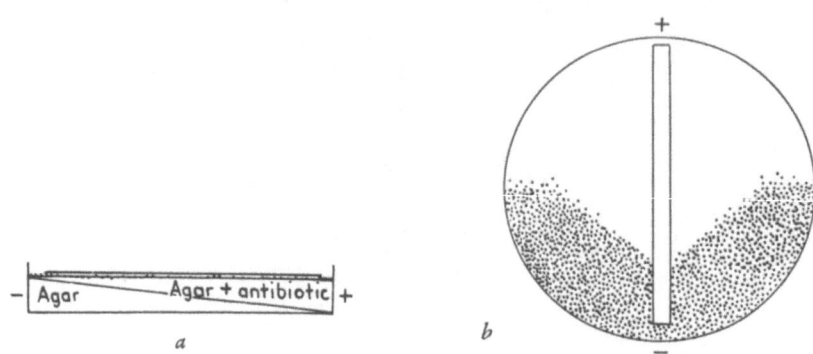

Fig. 3-14. Paper-strip-gradient test. (*a*) Agar layers in the plate. (*b*) Results of a positive test.

halfway down along the gradient. A suspension of bacteria is then spread on the surface of the plate, and after they have dried, a strip of filter paper soaked in the substance to be tested is placed on the surface of the plate at right angles to the gradient. If the substance has a potentiating effect, the kind of pattern shown in Fig. 3-14 *b* is observed.

In Fig. 3-14 the antibiotic in the medium is lankacidin, the potentiating substance in the strip is lankamycin, and the test organism is *S. aureus*. Under the conditions used, no inhibitory effect of lankamycin alone is detectable. This test is very sensitive to potentiating effects on antibiotic activity because of the linear concentration gradient of the antibiotic in the medium. On the other hand, quantitative evaluation of potentiating effects is difficult because the gradient of the potentiating substance is a logarithmic one, and it overlaps the linear gradient of the antibiotic.

One can also reverse the location of the components by putting the potentiating agent into the agar layer and by adding the inhibitor to the paper strip. For some situations this reversal of the components has an advantage in providing for greater sensitivity of the detection of a potentiating action.

This technique is not confined to testing potentiating agents but can be used in a more general manner to test for the effect of pH, ion concentration, etc. on the activity of an antibiotic.

The tests for antibiotic activity we have discussed so far in this chapter involve inhibition of growth of indicator strains. It should be pointed out that besides growth response other criteria can be used to test for antibiotic activity. For example, morphological changes in fungi may be valuable indicators of such an activity (see the "curling effect," p. 41). Another type of test involves inhibition of zygospore formation in *Mucor* without affecting growth of the organism. This type of test may reveal the existence of new types of antibiotics that cannot be detected by measuring growth response.

References

GROVE, D. C. and W. A. RANDALL, *Assay Methods of Antibiotics*, Antibiotic Monographs 2, Medical Encyclopedia, New York, 1955.

KAVANAGH, F., *Analytical Microbiology*, Academic Press, Inc., New York, 1963.

KLEIN, P., *Bakteriologische Grundlagen der Chemotherapeutischen Laboratoriumspraxis*. Springer, 1957.

MEYNELL, G. G. and E. MEYNELL, *Theory and Practice in Experimental Bacteriology*, 2d ed., Cambridge University Press, London, 1970.

Chapter 4

Biosynthesis

General Information

In the first chapter we considered the question of why antibiotics are synthesized. In this chapter we consider the question of how antibiotics are synthesized. These processes include the steps leading from the nutrients that are supplied to the cell to the end products. Besides its general value to our understanding of metabolism and its regulation such knowledge may have practical use. To illustrate this point, a biological precursor of an antibiotic may be easy to synthesize in the laboratory, whereas the finished product may present great difficulties. In such a case it may be possible to utilize the enzymatic machinery of the antibiotic-producing organism to accomplish the conversion of the synthetic precursor to the finished product.

Pathways of antibiotic synthesis are interwoven with pathways leading to primary metabolites, and investigation of antibiotic synthesis may therefore lead to the discovery of new intermediates in primary metabolism and to unexpected relationships among primary metabolic pathways. In this connection we should recall that the biosynthesis of antibiotics, like that of secondary metabolites in general, involves the following stages:

1. uptake of nutrients into the cell, and conversion to intermediates of the central metabolic routes (for example the glycolytic pathway, the Krebs citric acid cycle, the hexose monophosphate shunt);

2. a branching off into a pathway peculiar to the antibiotic after a number of steps via pathways of primary metabolism, which, besides the central intermediary routes, may involve biosynthetic pathways (for example amino acids, fatty acids, aromatic metabolites).

Among the branch-point reactions we may occasionally encounter unusual chemical reactions different from those of primary metabolism. Further conversions along the antibiotic-specific pathways are then carried out, leading to the final product. The overall picture that emerges is of a series of side branches leading off at various points from the network of primary metabolism.

The side branches may in themselves be quite complicated, involving the emergence of multiple branches from a given branch-point in primary metabolism or additional ramifications further down along the side branches. The reason for this complexity appears to be the tendency of an organism to form a whole series of secondary metabolites of a certain type once the capacity for carrying out the reactions leading into a particular secondary branch has been developed. This multiplicity may arise at the branch point from primary metabolism as a result of condensation of the primary metabolic intermediary with several substances initiating a series of side branches. It may also arise in the terminal portion of these branches by the shunting of a secondary intermediary product into a number of different directions. It is as though nature, once she had discovered a new pathway, were trying to explore all possible variations on a theme. It should be pointed out that this variety is not always readily recognized by the investigator, either because of lack of biological activity of some of the end products or because one end product is produced in such great preponderance that some of the minor components are overlooked. A few examples will illustrate this tendency toward multiplicity of related products.

1. Actinomycins. Each actinomycin-producing organism forms several actinomycins, all of which have the same phenoxazone chromophoric group but which differ from each other in their peptide chains.

2. Anthracyclines. *Streptomyces purpurascens* produces a large variety of rhodomycins, which differ from each other in the aglycone or in the sugar portion of the molecule. The same holds true for *Streptomyces galileus*, which produces pyrromycins.

3. Polymyxins. *Bacillus polymyxa* produces an almost unresolvable mixture of closely related peptide antibiotics.

This list could be extended by citing the macrolide antibiotics, the streptothricins, the purine antibiotics, and others. The production of mixtures of related substances occurs also among higher plants, for example in many related alkaloids produced by a single species.

One characteristic feature of secondary metabolites that distinguishes them from primary metabolites is frequent "uncontrolled" large-scale production by the organism. With the exception of a few vitamins, microorganisms do not produce primary metabolites (amino acids, purines, pyrimidines) in amounts greater than needed for growth. This economy is brought about mainly through metabolic regulatory mechanisms, especially enzyme induction, enzyme repression, and feedback inhibition. Accumulation of secondary metabolites suggests that the cells are inefficient in the regulation of synthesis of these substances. In view of what has been learned about the genetic control of regulation of primary metabolism it would be of interest to find out why the regulation of secondary metabolite formation is not controlled more strictly. By searching for mutants with either increased or decreased production of secondary metabolites and subsequent genetic analysis, one could find out whether or not there were specific regulatory genes, analogous to the regulatory genes of primary metabolism. This aspect of antibiotic biosynthesis has so far been studied relatively little, especially in regard to regulatory genes governing controls. In addition, as antibiotic synthesis is connected closely with primary metabolic pathways, and as these latter pathways are in many cases tightly controlled, it would be expected that control mechanisms functioning in primary metabolism also affect secondarily antibiotic biosynthesis.

The methods that have been generally used to elucidate biosynthetic pathways are isotopic tracer techniques, mutants blocked in such pathways, and demonstration of enzyme-catalyzed reactions. For antibiotic biosynthesis the first of these has been the most commonly used. With isotopes it is relatively easy to determine the origin of the building blocks of an antibiotic molecule, but it is more difficult to determine the nature of intermediates of a pathway. In the usual experiment the antibiotic-producing strain is grown with a given radioactive nutrient, the antibiotic is isolated, and the distribution of radioactivity in different parts of the antibiotic molecule is determined. In this type of procedure there are certain pitfalls, and results have to be interpreted cautiously. For example, because of many metabolic interconversions, presence of a specific grouping in an antibiotic molecule, also originally present in the labelled precursor substance, may nevero Originating from the methyl pool

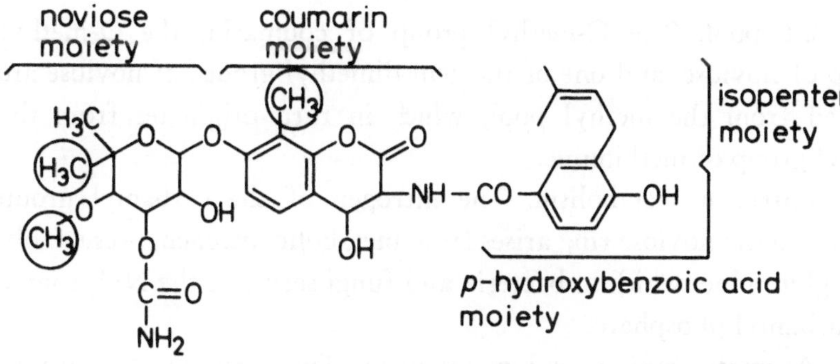

Fig. 4-1. Structure of novobiocin. Primary metabolic sources are indicated.

theless be caused by disruption of the original linkages and secondary reconstitution. In addition, since whole cells are employed in these experiments, failure of label to appear in an antibiotic molecule may be caused by impermeability of the cell to the labelled substance.

The following primary metabolic sources have been identified for those antibiotics whose synthesis is known or for which one has at least a plausible notion as to their metabolic origin:

1. fatty-acid metabolism (acetate and propionate);
2. amino-acid metabolism;
3. carbohydrate metabolism;
4. purine and pyrimidine metabolism;
5. aromatic biosynthesis (shikimic acid);
6. methyl groups arising from the C1 pool.

In the sections to follow we shall discuss each of these categories as a source of antibiotics. Before that, it should be made clear that many antibiotics originate from more than one of these metabolic sources. To dispel any notion of an obligatory single-source origin, we briefly consider the synthesis of novobiocin before proceeding with the discussion of the different metabolic sources, since this antibiotic clearly illustrates the origin of an antibiotic from a variety of metabolic sources.

Figure 4-1 shows the structure of novobiocin and the derivation of the different portions of the molecule. As can be seen, the building blocks are derived from the following metabolic sources:

1. Carbohydrate metabolism. The unbranched carbon chain of noviose is derived without cleavage from the carbon chain of glucose.

2. C1 pool. The C-methyl group of coumarin, the O-methyl group of noviose, and one of the gem-dimethyl groups of noviose are derived from the methyl pool, which in turn originates from the methyl group of methionine.

3. Nitrogen metabolism. The nitrogen of the carbamyl group attached to the noviose ring arises from metabolic nitrogen, presumably from glutamine, which in bacteria and fungi serves as the NH_2 source for carbamyl phosphate.

4. Aromatic amino acid metabolism. The 3-amino, 4-hydroxy-coumarin portion is derived from tyrosine, which in turn arises from the common aromatic pathway via shikimic acid.

5. Shikimic acid. The p-hydroxybenzoate portion is directly derived from the common aromatic pathway via shikimic acid, without prior passage through an aromatic amino acid.

6. Isopentyl metabolism. The isopentyl group attached to p-hydroxy-benzoate is derived from mevalonic acid, which in turn comes from either acetate or leucine.

Short-Chain Fatty Acids As Biosynthetic Precursors

Stepwise condensation of active acetate and malonate units (acetyl-CoA, malonyl-CoA) leads to the formation of β-polyketomethylene chains. Birch has demonstrated that by "head-tail" condensation of such units complicated natural products can be built up. The mechanism of β-polyketone synthesis was elucidated by Lynen and is shown schematically in Fig. 4-2. In this scheme a starter molecule of acetyl-CoA condenses with a molecule of malonyl-CoA to form acetoacetyl-CoA, with CO_2 being split off. The decarboxylation helps to drive the reaction in the forward direction. This assembly process does not occur freely in solution but is bound to an enzyme surface.

Substances that are biosynthetically derived from β-polyketones are called polyketides. Actually the starter molecule of polyketide synthesis is not always acetyl-CoA. It may be propionyl-CoA or more complicated CoA derivatives. For example, in the synthesis of tetra-cyclines the starter is malonamoyl-CoA (p. 46). Moreover, the units to be added to the starter are not always acetate units but may, for example, be propionate units, as in the synthesis of erythromycin (p. 43). As we mentioned above, the β-polyketone chains occur in the

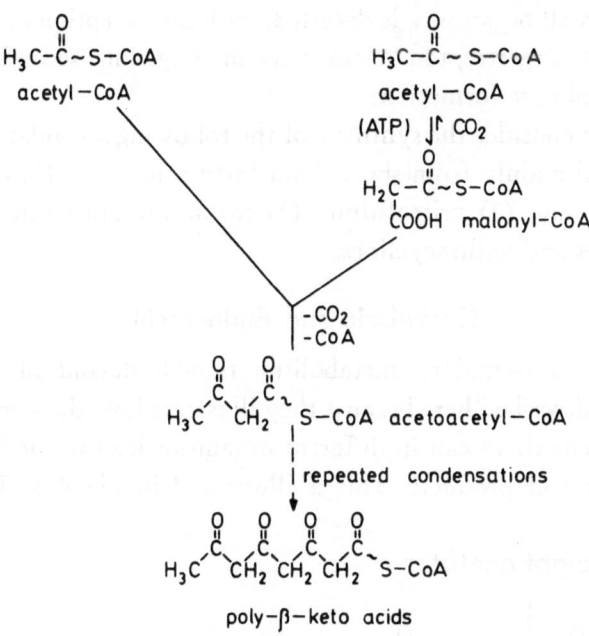

Fig. 4-2. Scheme of poly-β-keto acid synthesis.

cell as a rule bound to enzymes, and it has not been possible to trap them as free intermediates.

These intermediary β-polyketones undergo several types of further modifications. For example, reduction may lead to formation of fatty acids, which, however, does not occur in the formation of antibiotics. Introduction of double and triple bonds results in the formation of polyenes and polyacetylenes, the former being found in polyene antibiotics (nystatin, amphotericin, hamycin), which are widely distributed among actinomycetes, the latter being found among a variety of compounds occurring among basidiomycetes. Finally, cyclization leads to the formation of large lactones (macrolide antibiotics) or through repeated cyclization to polyaromatic compounds (tetracyclines, anthracyclines).

As we mentioned, β-polyketones are built up through head-tail condensation of acyl (mainly acetate) units. An exception is mevalonic acid, which though derived from acetate is not formed by head-tail condensation. It is also a precursor of a number of antibiotics but almost exclusively in fungi. It is surprising that this metabolite, which

is present in all organisms, is diverted, with the exception of the novo-
biocin-producing streptomycetes, only in fungi into secondary pathways of antibiotic formation.

We now consider the synthesis of the following secondary metabolites derived mainly from short-chain fatty acid units: (1) curvularin
and endocrocin, (2) griseofulvin, (3) macrolide antibiotics, and (4)
tetracyclines and anthracyclines.

Curvularin and Endocrocin

These two secondary metabolites, though devoid of antibiotic
action, are described here because they illustrate how the same β-poly-
ketomethylene chain can in different organisms lead to the formation
of different end products. This is illustrated in Fig. 4-3. The inter-

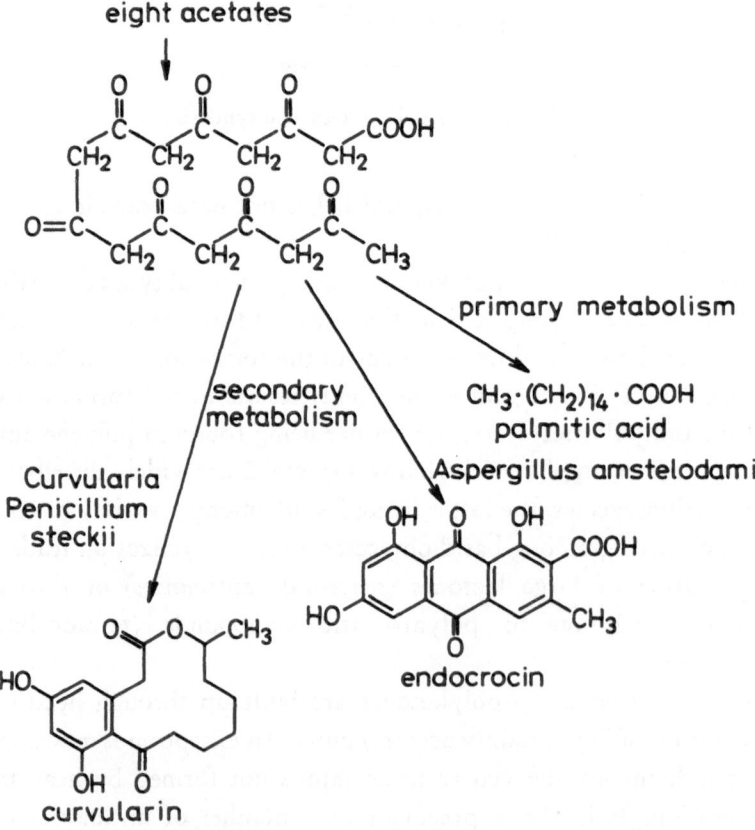

Fig. 4-3. Metabolic origins of curvularin and endocrocin.

mediary β-polyketone containing 16 carbon atoms is formed from eight acetate units. In primary metabolism this compound is reduced to form palmitic acid. In *Aspergillus amstelodami,* cyclization leads to the formation of the anthraquinone endocrocin, whereas in *Penicillium steckii* and a strain of *Curvularia,* cyclization is incomplete, resulting in the production of curvularin, which consists of an aromatic ring coupled to a lactone ring.

Griseofulvin

Figure 4-4 summarizes the biosynthesic pathway leading to griseofulvin. First a 14-carbon β-polyketomethylene chain is built up, which in primary metabolism would presumably be converted to myristic acid, a common constituent of fats. Many species of *Penicillium* are able to convert this intermediate to griseofulvin, employing a series of reactions consisting of cyclizations, methylations, and chlorinations. A compound not containing chlorine is also found among the fermentation products, but it has a much weaker antibiotic activity than griseofulvin.

Griseofulvin is an antifungal agent, being used in the treatment of dermatophytoses. At the lowest effective concentration it causes morphological changes in the hyphae ("curling effect") without, however, arresting growth. In order to inhibit growth completely a thousand times higher concentration of the antibiotic is required.

Erdin, a substance with a structure similar to griseofulvin is formed by *Aspergillus ferreus.* The pathway leading to griseofulvin or related substances is widespread among *Aspergillales,* but it is not found elsewhere.

Macrolide Antibiotics

Macrolide antibiotics are a group of substances obtained from *Streptomyces.* They contain a large lactone ring and one or more sugar residues. In most cases at least one of these sugars is a dimethylamino sugar. The sugars found are of an unusual nature (see Table 1-4). The following members of this group are therapeutically useful: carbomycin, erythromycin, leucomycin, oleandomycin, spiramycin, and tylosin. These constitute a small fraction of this class of compounds.

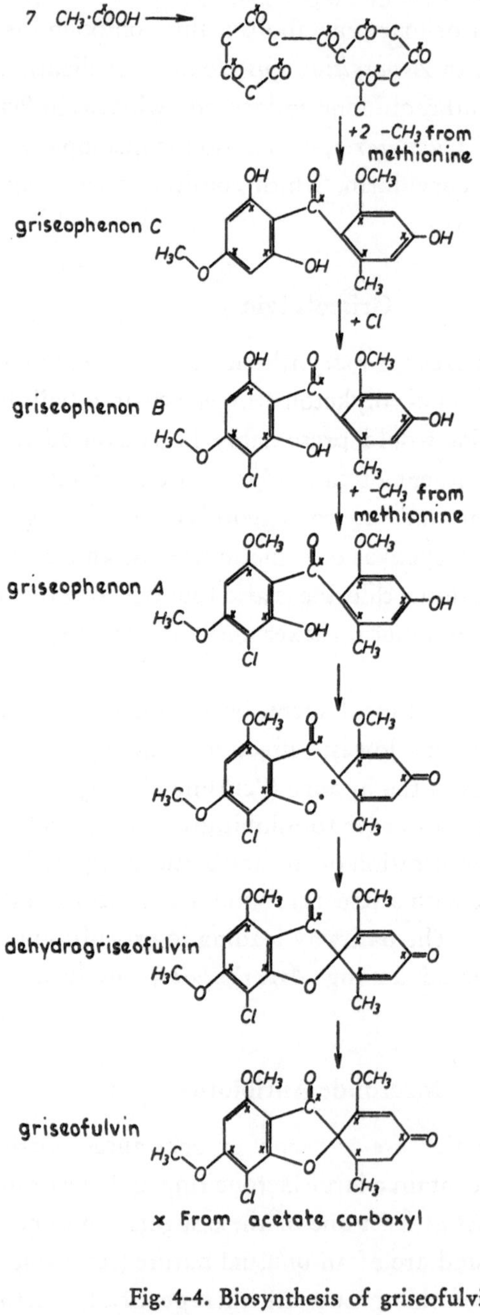

Fig. 4-4. Biosynthesis of griseofulvin.

At the present time macrolides are the largest group of well-characterized antibiotics.

The delineation of macrolides as a group is not clear cut. Several authors have assumed a broad enough definition to include the antifungal polyene antibiotics. These substances also contain a large lactone ring, and several of them contain a sugar residue. In addition, curvularin, rifamycin, and borrelidin may be thought of as "sugar-free macrolides." As we have seen (p. 40), in the case of curvularin and endocrocin two different substances may arise from the same β-polyketone intermediate, and in terms of biosynthetic origin there is no difference between the large lactone and the polycyclic compound. From these considerations it is clear that the macrolides are not as isolated and well-defined a group as they were thought to be originally.

The biosynthesis of macrolides has been successfully investigated mainly in the laboratories of Birch, Corcoran, and Grisebach. The lactone rings of these compounds are derived exclusively (erythromycin, methymycin) or predominantly (carbomycin) from short-chain fatty acids. Two types are found: those derived predominantly from propionate units (well-studied examples are erythromycin and methymycin) and those derived predominantly from acetate units (carbomycin). It may be assumed that this origin from short-chain fatty acids is also true for other, less thoroughly investigated macrolides.

Erythromycin. Figure 4-5 shows the origin of the carbon atoms of erythromycin. Seven propionate moieties participate in the formation of the lactone ring. Prior to the experimental demonstration of the origin from propionate there was disagreement about the source of these C3 units. Birch assumed an origin from acetate, with subsequent methylation. Woodward, on the other hand, postulated an origin directly from propionate or a similar C3 compound. Corcoran and Grisebach then demonstrated direct incorporation of propionate and could not find any incorporation of acetate.

Methymycin. The lactone ring of methymycin consists of five propionate units and one acetate unit (Fig. 4-6). Closely related in structure to this substance are pikromycin, griseomycin, and narbomycin, although the biosynthesis of these antibiotics has not yet been investigated. Like methymycin, these antibiotics contain one sugar,

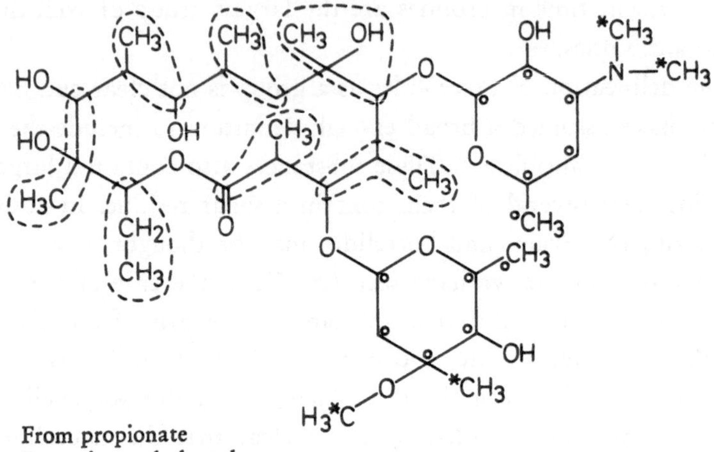

---- From propionate
 * From the methyl pool
 o From glucose, without cleavage

Fig. 4-5. Structure of erythromycin. Metabolic sources of the carbon skeleton are indicated.

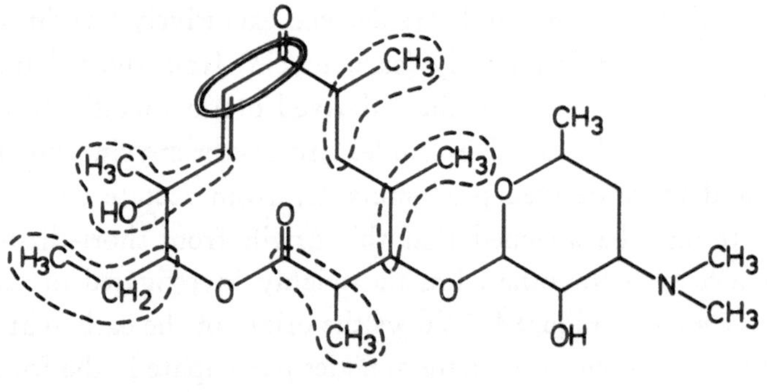

===== From acetate
---- From propionate

Fig. 4-6. Structure of methymycin, showing parts derived from acetate and from propionate.

desosamine. From their structures one may assume that picromycin is built up from five propionate units and one acetate unit, whereas in narbomycin there are six propionate units and one acetate unit.

Carbomycin. Figure 4-7 shows the origins of the complete carbon skeleton of carbomycin. Grisebach and coworkers, using C14-labelled precursors, have demonstrated origins from the following sources.

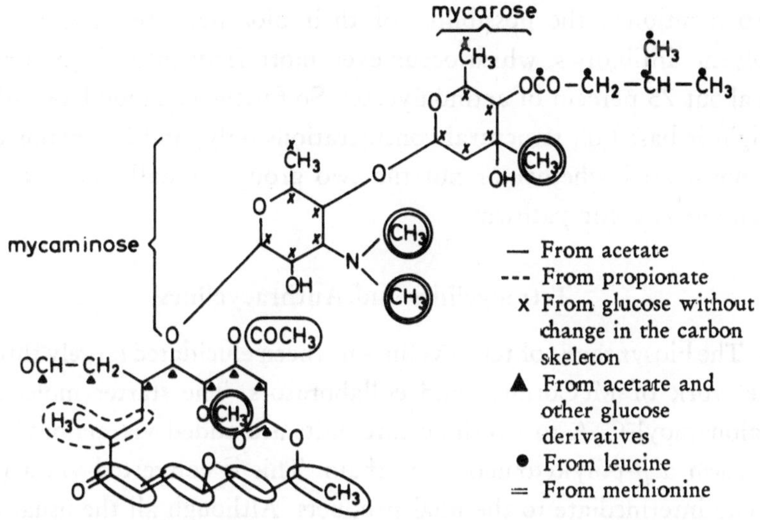

Fig. 4-7. Structure of carbomycin. Metabolic sources of the carbon skeleton are indicated.

Four acetate units are within the lactone ring, and one is attached to the lactone ring. In addition there is a C8 piece originating from acetate or pyruvate and another, so far unknown, precursor derived from glucose. One propionate unit is within the lactone ring. There are four methyl groups, derived from methionine, one attached to the lactone ring, the others forming part of the sugars. The isovalerate residue is derived from leucine. Finally the carbon skeletons of the two sugars are derived directly from glucose.

A few related macrolides may be mentioned: niddamycin (= desacetylcarbomycin), which presumably has the same biosynthetic derivation as carbomycin; acumycin, tylosin, and leucomycin resemble carbomycin both structurally and in their mode of action. We see that, as an illustration of our general scheme of antibiotic synthesis, the macrolide molecules are built from combinations of primary metabolites. It is not known now at which points the various components of the macrolide structures branch off from primary pathways nor how these components combine with each other into single compounds. As we have mentioned, among actinomycetes, macrolide antibiotics are distributed widely, being formed by 1 to 3 percent of all known strains. There is a great deal of variability in the structures found. We also mentioned the possibility of their biogenetic relationship with polyene antibiotics, which occur even more frequently, being present in about 75 percent of actinomycetes. So far the common biosynthetic origin is based on structural considerations only, and it remains to be demonstrated whether or not the two groups actually share a common biosynthetic pathway.

Tetracyclines and Anthracyclines

The biosynthesis of tetracyclines has been elucidated largely through the work of McCormick and collaborators. The starter molecule is malonamoyl-CoA to which acetate units are added via malonyl-CoA to form a β-polyketomethylene chain. This is converted via a polycyclic intermediate to the final products. Although all the usual techniques have been employed in working out this pathway, it was mainly the mutant methodology that was instrumental in this work. These mutants, like auxotrophs, lack an enzyme responsible for a given step of the pathway. One would expect accumulation of the substance before the genetic block, but here this is usually not the case. Instead the substance before the block undergoes the same series of reactions as the product of the affected reaction does in the wild type, thus leading to the formation of a modified end-product that lacks whatever the blocked reaction prevented from being added to the molecule. For example, a block in a methylating enzyme may lead to the same final product as that produced by the wild-type strain, except that it lacks a methyl group. A block between acetyl-CoA and malonamoyl-CoA leads to 2-acetyldecarboxamido tetracycline in which an acetyl group is substituted for the carbamyl group of tetracycline. Figure 4-8 shows a scheme for the biosynthesis of tetracycline and the products formed as a result of mutational blocks. The synthesis involves the following sequence of steps.

1. Synthesis of malonamoyl-CoA, blocked in mutant S6422. This mutant seems to have all the other enzymes of the pathway intact.
2. Formation of a β-polyketomethylene chain with the utilization of eight acetate units, via malonyl-CoA.
3. Methylation at C6, blocked in mutant S604. This mutant produces demethyltetracycline.

4. Ring closure, first of three rings, and subsequently of a fourth ring. The latter reaction is blocked in several mutants leading to three-ring aromatic products (protetrone).

5. Oxidation steps involving rings A and B. Here again mutants have been isolated that are partially or completely defective in these oxidations.

6. Chlorination at C7. In mutant S2308 this step is blocked leading to the formation of a dechlorinated product, whereas wild-type *S. aureofaciens* produces chlorotetracycline (aureomycin).

7. Amination at C4.

8. Methylation of the amino group at C4, the methyl groups arising from methionine.

9. Hydrogenation to form anhydrotetracycline. Mutants blocked in this step excrete metatrene, whose structure has not yet been established.

10. From anhydrotetracycline *S. rimosus* produces oxytetracycline via a not-yet elucidated intermediary compound.

11. From the same precursor *S. aureofaciens* can produce either chlorotetracycline, tetracycline, or 6-demethyltetracycline, according to what is substituted at C6 and C7. Mutants blocked in these reactions have been isolated that form 5-hydroxyanhydrotetracycline or tetramide blue.

In Fig. 4-8 the structures of those postulated intermediates that have not been elucidated are put in parentheses. It has already been pointed out that the intracellular concentration of intermediates is low and that in many instances they remain bound to a multienzyme complex.

Four-ring systems are also found in anthracycline antibiotics. The aglycones of these substances can be derived from β-polyketones. For ε-pyrromycinone, which is identical with the aglycone portion of pyrromycin, cinerubines and rubilantin, the origin from one propionate unit and nine acetate units has been demonstrated by Ollis (Fig. 4-9). All anthracyclines contain in addition to the anthracyclinone portion one or several sugars, including dimethylaminosugars. These sugars are chemically similar to those found in macrolide antibiotics. In fact the structural relationship between these two groups extends not only to the sugars but also to the aglycone portion, and one can

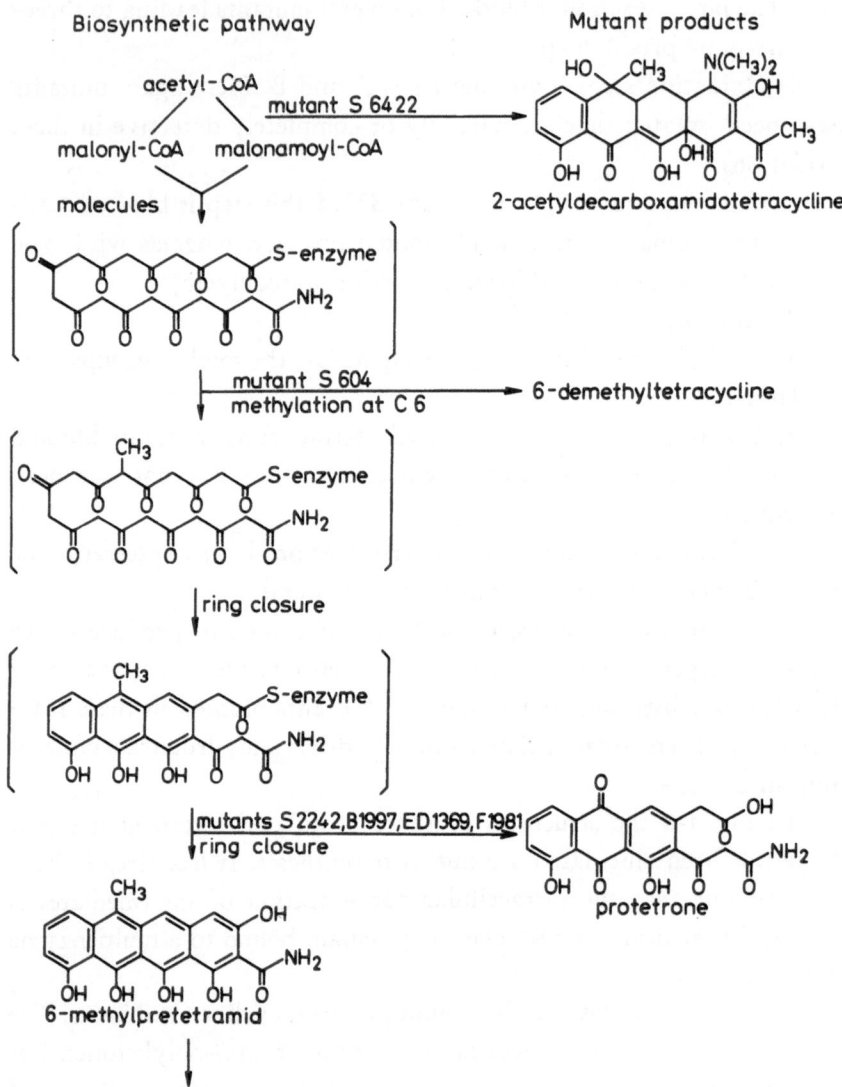

Fig. 4-8. Scheme of tetracycline synthesis, with mutational blocks and mutant products indicated. (According to McCormick, see Gottlieb, D. and P. D. Shaw, eds.; "Antibiotics. II. Biosynthesis", Springer-Verlag, New York, 1967.

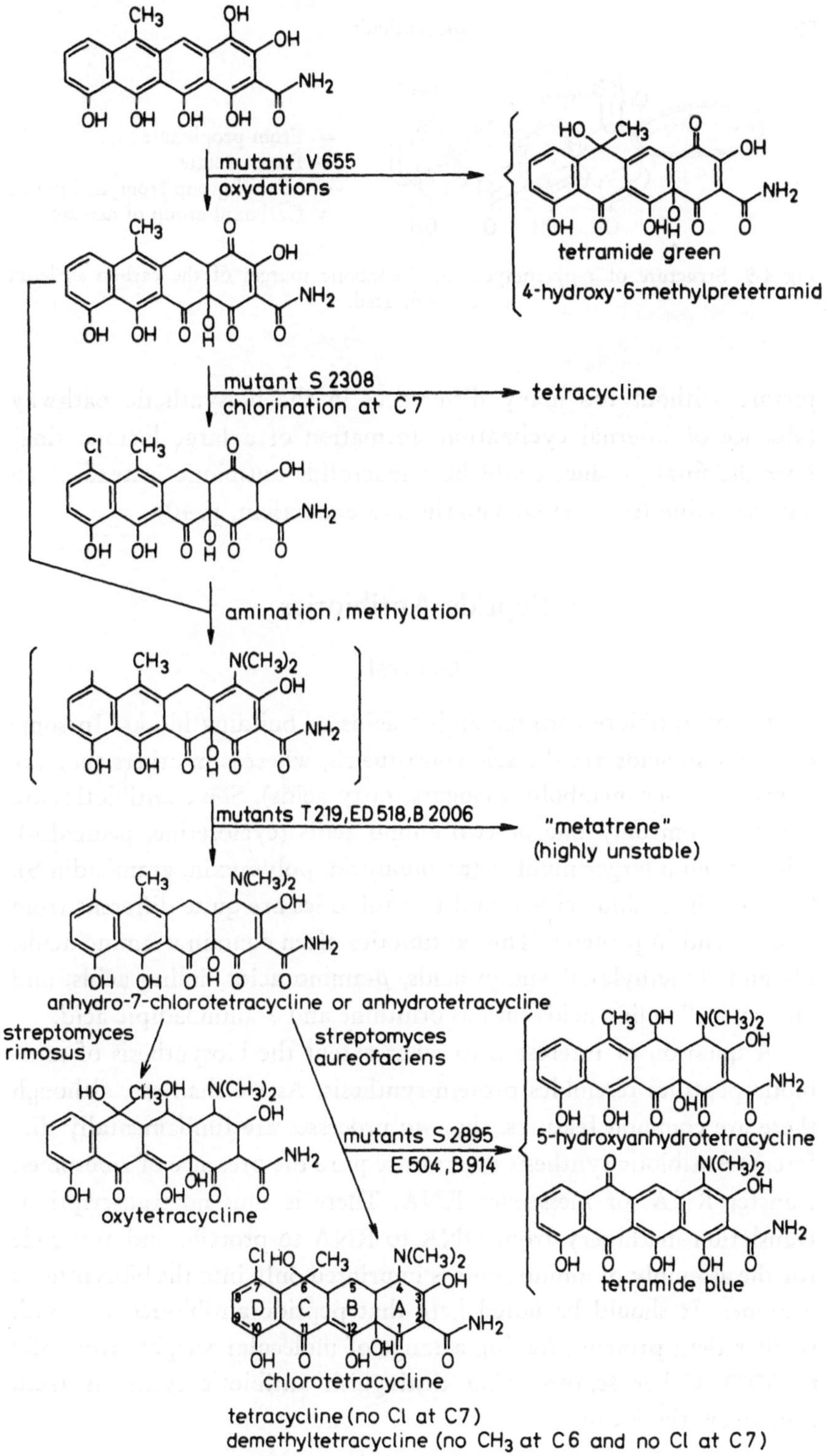

mutant V 655
oxydations

tetramide green
4-hydroxy-6-methylpretetramid

mutant S 2308
chlorination at C 7 → tetracycline

amination, methylation

mutants T 219, ED 518, B 2006 → "metatrene"
(highly unstable)

anhydro-7-chlorotetracycline or anhydrotetracycline

streptomyces rimosus

streptomyces aureofaciens

mutants S 2895
E 504, B 914

5-hydroxyanhydrotetracycline

tetramide blue

oxytetracycline

chlorotetracycline

tetracycline (no Cl at C7)
demethyltetracycline (no CH₃ at C6 and no Cl at C7)

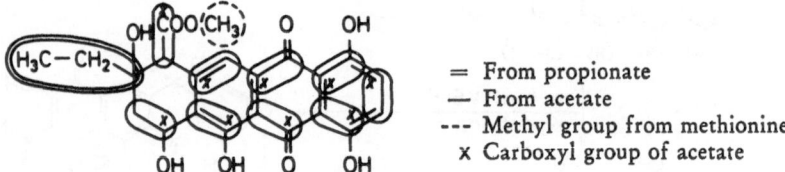

Fig. 4-9. Structure of ε-pyrromycinone. Metabolic sources of the carbon skeleton are indicated.

picture without too many differences in the biosynthetic pathway (absence of internal cyclization, formation of a large lactone ring) how the final product could be a macrolide antibiotic instead of an anthracycline (see also curvularin and endocricin, p. 40).

Peptide Antibiotics

General

Many antibiotics utilize amino acids as building blocks. In some cases amino acids are the sole constituents, whereas in others they are joined to other metabolites (sugars, fatty acids). Some antibiotics are derived from only one or two amino acids (cycloserine, penicillin), others from a larger number (actinomycin, polymyxin, gramicidin S). Some of the amino acids found in antibiotics are quite different from those found in proteins. Thus antibiotics often contain D-amino acids, N- and β-methylated amino acids, β-amino acids, imino acids, and "precursor" amino acids such as ornithine and α-aminoadipic acid.

A question of interest is to what extent the biosynthesis of antibiotic peptides resembles protein synthesis. As we shall see, although there are common features, the two processes are fundamentally different. Antibiotic synthesis does not require the presence of ribosomes, transfer RNA, or messenger RNA. There is thus no transcription-translation machinery from DNA to RNA to protein, and any code for the assembly of amino acids is imprinted only into the biosynthetic enzymes. It should be noted here that peptide antibiotics are much smaller than proteins, having a range of molecular weights from 350 to 3000. Other features that distinguish antibiotic synthesis from protein synthesis are

Table 4-1 Some Polypeptide Antibiotics

Name and producing organism	"Usual" amino acids	"Unusual" amino acids	Other component
Gramicidin S *Bacillus brevis*	2 L-Val 2 L-Leu 2 L-Pro	2 L-Orn 2 D-Phe —	— —
Bacitracin *Bacillus licheniformis*	12 L-Ile 1 L-Leu 1 L-Asp 1 L-Lys 1 L-His	1 D-Glu 1 D-Asp-NH_2 1 D-Orn 1 D-Phe	Thiazoline moiety (from L-Cys and L-Ile)
Edeine *Bacillus brevis*	1 Gly —	iso-Ser iso-Tyr α,β-Diaminopropionic acid 2,6-Diamino-7-hydroxy-azaleic acid	Spermidine —
Polymyxin B₁ *Bacillus polymyxa*	2 L-Thr 1 L-Leu	1 D-Phe 6 L-Diaminobutyric acid	(+)-6-Methyl-octanoate —
Actinomycin D (IV) *Streptomyces antibioticus*	2 L-Thr 2 L-Pro	2 D-Val 2 Sarcosine 2 N-methyl-valine	Phenozazin-one —
Echinomycin *Streptomyces echinatus*	2 L-Ala —	2 D-Ser 2 N-methyl-valine	2-Quinoxaline Carboxylic acid Dithiane ring
Etamycin *Streptomyces lavendulae*	1 L-Thr 1 L-Ala	1 D-Leu 1 D-Allo-hydroxyproline 1 Sarcosine 1 α-Phenylsarcosine 1 N,β-dimethyl-L-leucine	3-Hydroxy-picolinic acid —

1. relaxation in the specificity of assembly resulting usually in the production of a family of closely related substances rather than a unique polypeptide chain;

2. formation of cyclic structures with no free α-amino or α-carboxyl groups;

3. insensitivity to protein-synthesis inhibitors such as chloramphenicol and puromycin;

4. *in vivo* production during a late stage of the growth cycle, after protein synthesis has ceased. In the case of sporulating bacilli, antibiotic production seems to be associated with the process of sporulation.

In the following sections we consider the synthesis of two representative antibiotics, penicillin (and cephalosporin), and gramicidin S, mainly to illustrate what has been learned about the principles underlying the formation of peptide antibiotics. Table 4-1 lists a number of peptide antibiotics of medical and other interest, and shows their constituent amino acids and other building blocks.

Penicillin and Cephalosporin

Penicillin is the most important antibiotic medically, and for this reason alone it deserves careful consideration. There are actually a number of penicillins, all of which have the same β-lactone-thiazolidine ring system, but they differ fom each other in the nature of their side chains. One of the most effective and widely used penicillins is penicillin G, which has a phenylacetyl side chain. Metabolically the ring system is derived from L-valine and L-cysteine. During the biosynthesis of penicillin, L-α-Aminoadipic acid condenses in stepwise fashion with these two amino acids to form a tripeptide. L-Cysteine and L-valine undergo a series of internal condensations to form two rings, after which the aminoadipyl side chain is replaced by another side chain. This series of reactions starting from the amino acid (primary metabolite) precursors is shown in Fig. 4-10. L-α-Aminoadipic acid, a precursor of L-lysine, condenses with L-cysteine to form the corresponding dipeptide, which in turn reacts with L-valine to form the corresponding tripeptide. In the next step dehydrogenation results in the formation of a β-lactam ring. A further dehydrogenation at the valine α- and β-carbons results in the loss of optical activity of the valine moiety, and provides the substrate for ring closure to form the thiazolidine ring, with inversion of configuration at the valine α-carbon atom. This substance is isopenicillin N. The next step, yet to be firmly established experimentally, is an exchange reaction of the aminoadipyl side chain with another carboxylic acid catalyzed by a transferase. For example, exchange with phenylacetic acid forms penicillin G. In the absence of an acceptor, the side chain may be split off by an acylase to produce 6-aminopenicillanic acid. This latter compound is an important starting material for the formation of "semisynthetic" penicillins. Figure 4-10 also shows the synthesis of the closely related cephalosporin C, to which we shall come shortly.

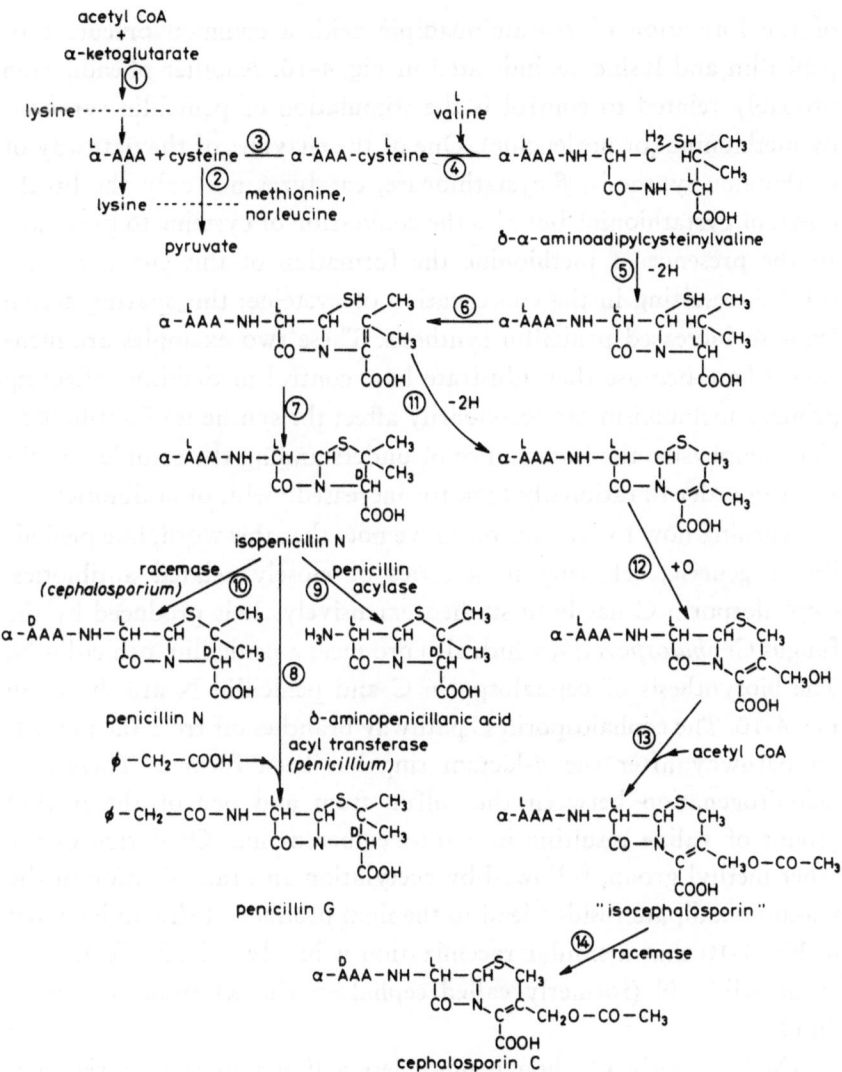

Fig. 4-10. Hypothetical pathway for the biosynthesis of penicillin G, penicillin N, and cephalosporin C. Dotted lines indicate inhibition. Abbreviations: α-aminoadipic acid, α-AAA; phenyl Φ; coenzyme A, CoA. (From A. L. Demain in J. F. Snell, ed., *Biosynthesis of Antibiotics*, Academic Press, 1966.)

A few points may be noted about the control of this biosynthetic pathway. It was found a long time ago by Bonner that some lysine-requiring mutants of *P. notatum* failed to produce penicillin, and later Demain showed that lysine was an inhibitor of penicillin synthesis in *P. chrysogenum*. This can be explained by feedback inhibition of the formation of L-α-aminoadipic acid, a common precursor of penicillin and lysine, as indicated in Fig. 4-10. Another phenomenon probably related to control is the stimulation of penicillin synthesis by methionine (or norleucine). One of the enzymes of the pathway of methionine synthesis, β-cystathionase, catalyzes not only the breakdown of cystathionine but also the conversion of cysteine to pyruvate. In the presence of methionine the formation of this enzyme is repressed, resulting in the conservation of cysteine; this sparing action leads to increased penicillin synthesis. These two examples are mentioned here because they illustrate how control mechanisms affecting primary metabolism can secondarily affect the synthesis of antibiotics. They emphasize the importance of understanding the complete pathways in order to rationally look for increased yields of antibiotics.

Turning now to cephalosporin we note that this word, like penicillin, is generic, referring to a series of closely related antibiotics. Cephalosporin C has been studied extensively. It is produced by the fungus *Cephalosporium,* which also produces a penicillin, penicillin N. The biosynthesis of cephalosporin C and penicillin N are shown in Fig. 4-10. The cephalosporin C pathway branches off from the penicillin pathway after the β-lactam ring has been formed. There is a dehydrogenation between the sulfur atom and one of the methyl groups of valine resulting in a six-membered ring. Oxidation of the other methyl group, followed by acetylation and racemization of the L-α-aminoadipate residue lead to the final product. It should be noted in Fig. 4-10 that a similar racemization is involved in the formation of penicillin N (formerly called cephalosporin N) from isopenicillin N.

Cephalosporin C, though much less active against bacteria than penicillin G, and of little medical usefulness, has certain properties that have preserved interest in this compound from a therapeutic point of view. Thus it is relatively insensitive to penicillinase (β-lactamase) and has a broader antibacterial spectrum than penicillin G. It has been possible to chemically replace the aminoadipate side chain with other side chains, as has been done with penicillin, and in this way much more effective compounds have been obtained, analogous to the semisynthetic penicillins. For example, replacement by phenylacetic acid results in a 100-fold increase of activity. This increase is similar to that observed when the aminoadipyl side chain on penicillin N is replaced by a phenylacetyl side chain to give penicillin G. A number of therapeutically useful cephalosporins have been developed in this fashion (cephalorin and cephaloridine, for instance), which besides being resistant to β-lactamase action, have the additional advantage of not being cross-allergenic with penicillin.

Gramicidin S

This antibiotic has been chosen because the mechanism of assembly from the amino-acid level has been elucidated by studies with a cell-free enzyme system. The structure of gramicidin S is shown in Fig. 4-11. It is a cyclic decapeptide, consisting of two identical pentapeptide units. It is produced by certain strains of *B. brevis*.

The cell-free system has been studied by Kleinkauf and Gevers in F. Lipmann's laboratory, and it consists of two protein fractions, I and II. These fractions have been purified about 100-fold. The sequence of steps postulated by these workers is shown in Fig. 4-11. The first step is the formation of an enzyme-bound adenylate from ATP and the amino acid, similar to the activation of amino acids for protein synthesis. Fraction I (presumably a multienzyme complex) catalyzes the activation of four L-amino acids, whereas fraction II catalyzes the activation of L-phenylalanine, followed by racemization. In the next reaction a transfer occurs from the adenylate to a SH group on the surface of the enzymes. Conditions are now set for initiation of peptide-bond formation. The first peptide bond is formed between D-phenylalanine and L-proline, and it involves transfer of the phenylalanyl residue from fraction II to the amino group of L-proline. Further elongation occurs in a fixed order by transfer reactions within fraction I, with the activated carboxyl group of the growing peptide chain being transferred to the amino group of the activated amino acid. The last amino acid to be added to the chain is L-leucine. At this point the finished decapeptide is formed, presumably by an antiparallel coupling reaction between two carboxyl-activated pentapeptidyl units, as shown in Fig. 4-11.

The overall reaction thus resembles protein synthesis in regard to formation of an enzyme-bound adenylate, the direction of chain

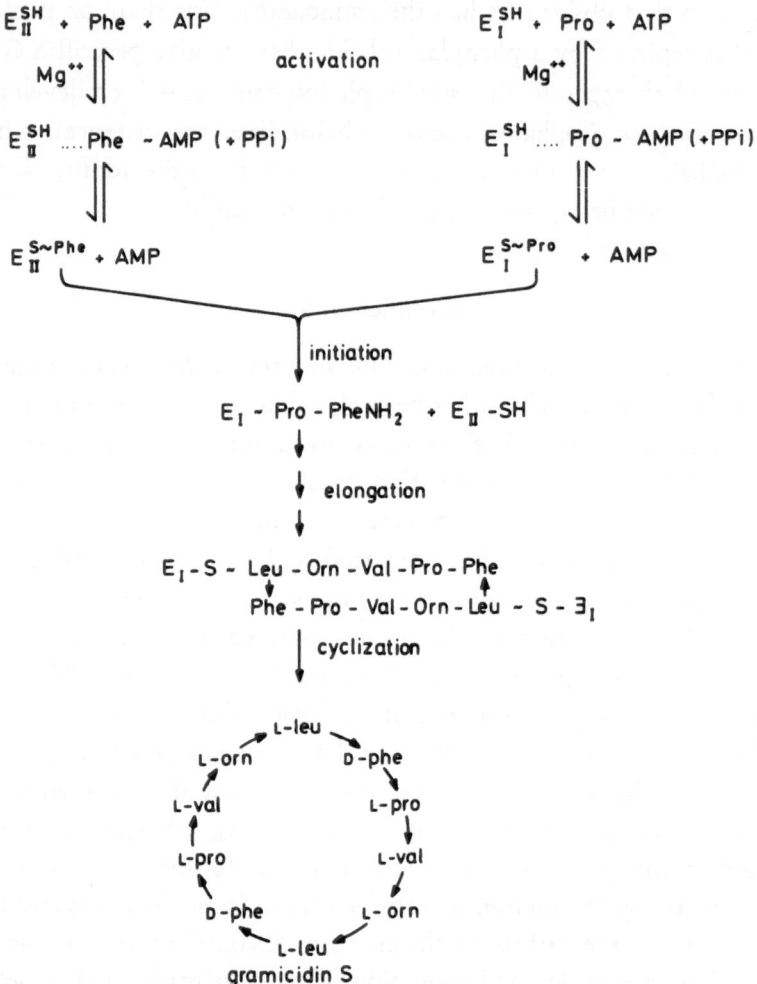

Fig. 4-11. Scheme of the enzymatic synthesis of gramicidin S. (Modified from Kleinkauf and Gevers.)

growth, and the retention of a carboxyl-activated intermediate until
the final splitting off of the finished product. It differs from protein
synthesis in that enzyme SH groups rather than an adapter transfer
RNA act as acceptors after the primary activation. The sequence of
amino acids in gramicidin S is determined by a unique arrangement
of specific enzymes in a multienzyme complex rather than the sequence of triplets on a messenger RNA, and this imposes much greater
limitations on the size of the peptide that can be produced. It also

results in a less faithful translation of the information than is found in protein synthesis, as shown by the much greater chance for amino-acid substitutions ("ambiguity") found with gramicidin S and peptide antibiotics in general, than with proteins.

The type of mechanism depicted here represents an intermediate stage of complexity between the assembly reactions of proteins and other template-directed macromolecules and the simple enzyme-catalyzed reactions of intermediary metabolism. One may ask whether the assembly process illustrated by the synthesis of gramicidin S represents a primitive stage in the evolution of the protein-bio-synthetic machinery, or alternatively, an offshoot type of mechanism that, because of inherent limitations, could not lead to further evo-lutionary developments. The answer to this question is not known. The question has a bearing on the role of nucleic acids in the origin of life and the stage of evolution at which nucleic acids became essen-tial parts of living cells.

Sugars as Constituents of Antibiotics

We shall confine ourselves to a few remarks concerning three major points.

1. Sugars occur widely among antibiotics produced by actino-mycetes. An impression of the variety of sugars present may be gained from Table 1-4, which lists some of the sugars present in macrolide antibiotics. Other groups of antibiotics that contain sugars include aminoglycoside antibiotics (streptomycin, kanamycin, neomycin, and others), anthracyclines, purine-antibiotics (puromycin, for example), and polyene-antibiotics (nystatin, amphoterin, and others).

Among fungal antibiotics the occurrence of sugar moieties is rare. It is especially noteworthy that no sugar-containing antibiotics have been found among *Aspergillales*. Among Bacilli, also, no sugar-con-taining antibiotics have been found, the majority being peptide anti-biotics.

2. As already mentioned, many of the sugars present in actino-mycete-antibiotics are limited to actinomycetes and do not occur in other groups of organisms.

3. A large fraction of the sugars present in actinomycete-antibiotics are amino sugars, about one-third of these sugars having been found to contain nitrogen. Little is known about the biosynthesis of these sugars. The following statements can be made, based mainly on work with macrolide sugars: (1) the carbon skeleton of unbranched sugars is derived directly from glucose and (2) in branched sugars C-methyl groups are derived from the methyl pool, presumably from methionine, whereas the remaining carbon chain is derived from glucose. The N-methyl group of dimethylamino sugars also comes from the methyl pool. It may be noted here that in streptomycin the C-formyl group of streptose originates from the C3 atom of glucose by a rearrangement of the carbon chain. (For the formula of streptomycin see p. 109.)

Antibiotics Containing Purines or Pyrimidines

A number of antibiotics are known that are analogs of purine ribosides, the modification from the normal metabolite being present either in the purine ring, in the sugar moiety, or in both. The antibiotics to be described are derived from adenine mononucleotide (AMP), and their structures are shown in Fig. 4-12 *a* and *b*. Modification of the sugar moiety is found in cordycepin, psicofuranine, and angustmycin A. In cordycepin (produced by two fungi, *Cordyceps militaris* and *Aspergillus nidulans*) the conversion of ribose to 3-deoxyribose occurs at the level of "bound ribose" either in adenosine or AMP; that is, the antibiotic is a conversion product of AMP. In psicofuranine, synthesis involves the replacement of the ribose moiety of AMP by the 6-carbon sugar D-psicose (D-allulose), which is derived from glucose. Angustmycin A can be formed *in vivo* directly from psicofuranine by oxidation at carbon atom five of the sugar, and since both antibiotics are produced by the same organism *(Streptomyces hygroscopicus)* it seems likely that psicofuranine is formed first and that angustmycin A is derived from it.

Modification of the purine-ring structure is seen in nebularin, tubercidin, and toyocamycin. Of the three, nebularin bears the closest resemblance to adenosine. In the other two the nitrogen in position

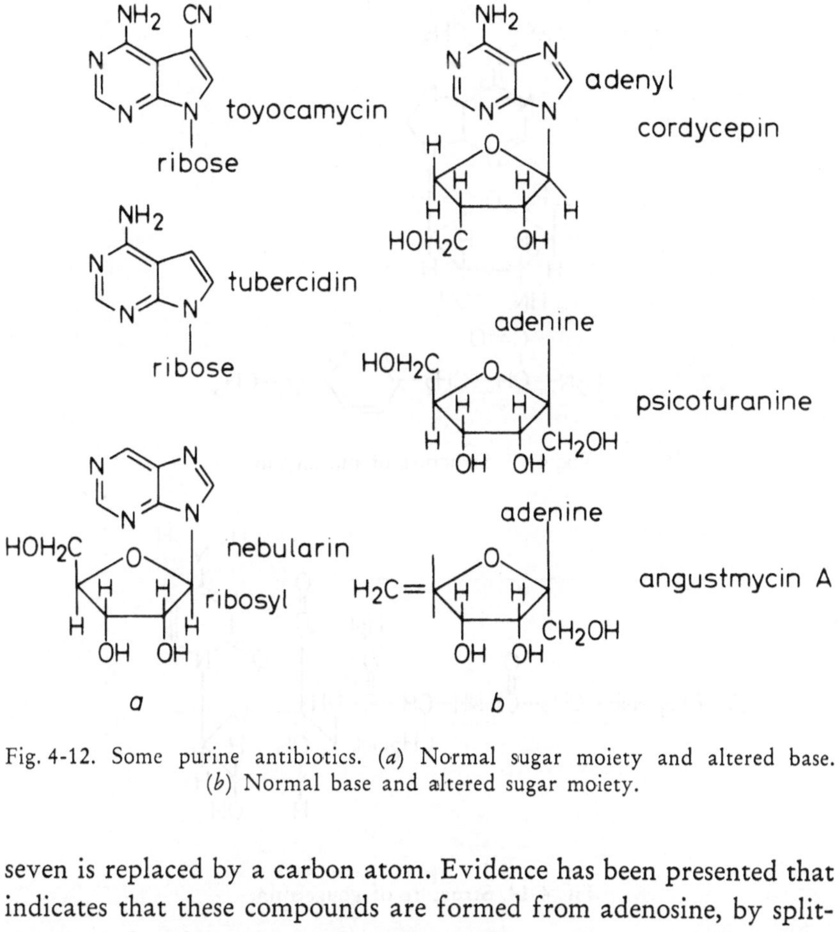

Fig. 4-12. Some purine antibiotics. (a) Normal sugar moiety and altered base. (b) Normal base and altered sugar moiety.

seven is replaced by a carbon atom. Evidence has been presented that indicates that these compounds are formed from adenosine, by splitting out of carbon atom eight and nitrogen atom seven, followed by reaction with PRPP from which the two-ring carbons are derived. The carbon of the cyano group of toyocamycin, a rare group among biological compounds, is also derived from ribose.

A purine antibiotic with modifications in the sugar and the purine ring is puromycin (Fig. 4-13). This compounds contains dimethyl adenine and ribosamine linked to O-methyl tyrosine. It has been used widely in studies on protein synthesis, and we shall return to it in the next chapter.

A small number of pyrimidine antibiotics has been described. One of these, gougerotin (Fig. 4-14) is structurally similar to puromycin. Both of them may be considered as analogs of the amino-acid binding end of transfer RNA; and both of them act in a similar way in protein

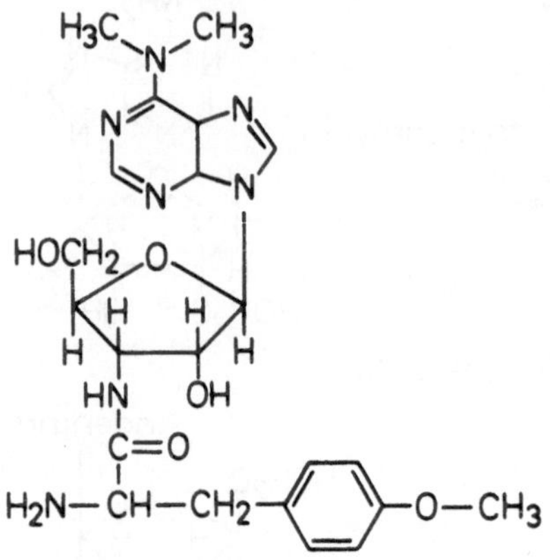

Fig. 4-13. Structure of puromycin.

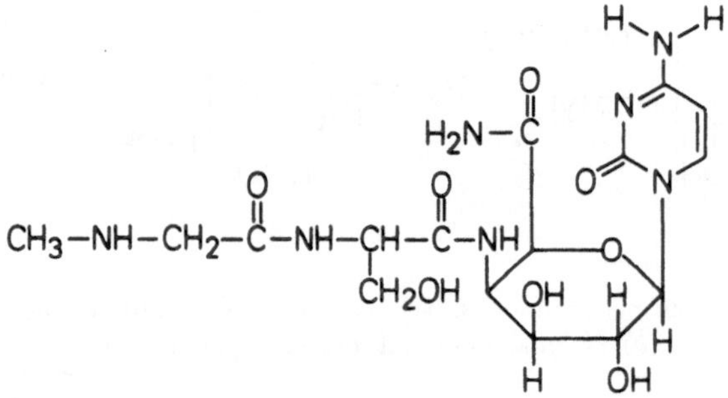

Fig. 4-14. Structure of gougerotin.

synthesis. In puromycin the purine moiety may be thought of as being derived from adenine, whereas in gougerotin the pyrimidine moiety may be thought of as coming from cytosine.

Derivatives of Shikimic Acid

Shikimic acid is a key intermediate in the biosynthesis of aromatic amino acids and other metabolites (*p*-aminobenzoic acid, *p*-hydroxy-benzoic acid, ubiquinone, and others). In higher plants it is also the source of many secondary metabolites (coumarins, phenols, lignins, flavonoids, and others). Surprisingly, among microorganisms, there are relatively few secondary metabolites derived from shikimic acid. Novobiocin (see Fig. 4-1) may be cited as an example of an antibiotic derived partly from the aromatic pathway.

References

BIRKINSHAW, J. H., "Chemical Constituents of the Fungal Cell. Special Chemical Products," in C. C. AINSWORTH and A. S. SUSSMAN, *The Fungi*, vol. I, Academic Press, Inc. New York, 1965.

BU'LOCK, J. D., *The Biosynthesis of Natural Products*, McGraw-Hill, Inc. London, 1965.

GOTTLIEB, D. and P. D. SHAW, eds., "Antibiotics. II. *Biosynthesis*," Springer-Verlag, New York, 1967.

KLEINKAUF, H. and W. GEVERS, "Nonribosomal polypeptide synthesis: The biosynthesis of a cyclic peptide antibiotic, gramicidin S," *Cold Spring Harbor Symp. Quant. Biol.* 34, 805–813, 1969.

VANEK, Z. and Z. HOSTALEK, eds., *Biogenesis of Antibiotic Substances*, Academic Press, Inc. New York, 1965.

WHALLEY, W. B., "The Biosynthesis of Fungal Metabolites," in B. BERNFELD, *Biogenesis of Natural Compounds*, Pergamon Press, Inc. London, 1963.

Chapter 5

Mode of Action

General Information

Antibiotics inhibit growth either reversibly (bacteristatic) or irreversibly (bactericidal). This inhibition is a result of interference with reactions that are essential for growth. Such reactions may be in the biosynthetic pathways leading to metabolic building blocks or coenzymes, in the synthesis of macromolecules, such as proteins and nucleic acids, or in the maintenance and synthesis of cellular structures, such as the cell wall or the cell membrane. To determine the mode of action of an antibiotic is to find out first the reaction whose inhibition is responsible for the observed inhibition of growth and then to find the way in which the antibiotic blocks that particular reaction.

A given antibiotic may inhibit several reactions, and the number of reactions inhibited may depend on its concentration in the testing medium. The reactions blocked may be either essential or not essential for growth. With an antibiotic affecting several reactions as the concentration of the antibiotic is increased, more and more reactions may be affected. This dependence on concentration presumably reflects differences in the sensitivity of different reactions toward the inhibitor and in most cases results from differences in the affinities of affected enzymes. Furthermore, the blocking of one reaction may secondarily lead to inhibition of other reactions, this being another way in which an antibiotic may affect several reactions. The somewhat confusing array of actions that an antibiotic may have can be illustrated by the example of streptomycin. Without going into details at this time, this drug affects protein synthesis, RNA and DNA synthesis, the integrity of the cell membrane, and respiration, and it is not always possible to distinguish in this case between separate primary effects on different reactions and secondary effects produced on a reaction as a result of interference with another reaction. To find out the mode of action in such a case is to discover the reaction or reactions *primarily* affected by the drug that are essential for growth.

It may be instructive to list some of the difficulties and limitations encountered in the elucidation of the mode of action of an antibiotic.

1. As can be seen from the previous discussion, in whole cells it is difficult to tell primary effects apart from secondary effects, and it therefore becomes necessary to attempt this by testing the effect of the antibiotics in cell-free systems. This may also be difficult, especially with systems of macromolecular synthesis and with structural elements.

2. Antibiotics are for the most part complicated chemical substances, and it is often impossible to synthesize them chemically. This means that they have to be obtained through fermentation procedures, which may create limitations in certain situations, as for example in obtaining radioactive compounds of high specific activity or in obtaining structural analogs of the antibiotic. Both kinds of compounds are valuable tools in exploring the mode of action of an antibiotic.

3. The essential reaction blocked by an antibiotic may be in an area not well understood biochemically, and it may then be impossible to localize the reaction affected. As we shall see, this is a difficulty in considering effects on protein synthesis. It also holds true, more or less, for other macromolecular syntheses — least for the synthesis of the mucopeptide component of cell walls.

4. Organisms differ from each other in their metabolism, and what may be determined as the mode of action in one organism may not be the way in which the antibiotic inhibits growth in most other organisms.

We next enumerate some of the methods used in investigating the mode of action of an antibiotic. None of these methods alone permits a determination of the mode of action with certainty, and it is only through combination of several of these methods that a definitive answer can be obtained.

Binding of the Antibiotic to Its Site of Action. The antibiotic has to combine with its target site in order to act, and if the binding is tight it may be detected with a radioactive antibiotic with high specific activity. For example, penicillin-sensitive organisms bind S^{35}-penicillin, and this binding occurs in the cytoplasmic membrane. Experiments with fluorescence-labelled polymyxin (1-dimethylamino-naphthalene-5-sulfonamido-polymyxin) suggested binding to the cellular phospholipid fraction. C^{14}-streptomycin is bound to ribosomes obtained from sensitive, but not from resistant, organisms.

A limitation of this method is that for some antibiotics there are only a few binding sites per cell, so that a very high specific activity is required to demonstrate labelling of these sites and to avoid confusion caused by binding at other sites, which may occur as the concentration of labelled antibiotic is increased. Streptomycin, for example, being a basic compound, binds nonspecifically to many acidic substances, especially nucleic acids, and it can be used at elevated concentrations in the purification of enzymes to precipitate nucleic acids and to separate them from proteins.

Effect of the Antibiotic on Specific Enzymatic Reactions. This method can give a clear-cut answer in regard to the mode of action, provided that the enzymatic reaction affected by an antibiotic can be localized. Without prior indications for possible sites of action from other studies this is a hopeless task. If, however, the mode of action of an antibiotic has previously been narrowed down to a given pathway and if the enzymes of that pathway can be studied in cell-free extracts, then one can find out not only which enzyme is affected but also the nature of the inhibition, such as competition with the substrate, allosteric inhibition, noncompetitive inhibition, and so on,

Accumulation of Substances in the Presence of an Antibiotic. A block in a biosynthetic sequence $A \rightleftharpoons B \rightleftharpoons C$ may lead to the accumulation of the substrate of the blocked reaction (B) or even earlier precursors in the chain. Whether or not the immediate precursor or earlier precursors will be accumulated depends among other things on the equilibrium constants of the reactions before the block. This method presupposes that there are no branches before the block that convert precursors to other end products. It should also be kept in mind that a block resulting from a secondary effect of the antibiotic may also lead to the accumulation of precursors.

Techniques that are useful in the detection and characterization of accumulated precursors are paper chromatography and thin-layer chromatography. With both methods, accumulated compounds may be detected by using the growth response of a microorganism for which the accumulated substance is a growth factor (bioautography). An example of the usefulness of the chromatographic method is the demonstration of the accumulation of UDP-muramyl peptides ("Park compounds") in the presence of penicillin. This finding was one of the earliest indications that penicillin inhibits cell-wall synthesis.

Agents That Reverse the Inhibition Caused by the Antibiotic. In our hypothetical example of a block in a biosynthetic sequence $A \rightleftharpoons B \rightleftharpoons C \rightleftharpoons D$ the inhibition of growth resulting from the block between B and C can be reversed by the addition of C or D, and in the case of competitive inhibition, by an excess of B. Thus the finding of reversing agents may provide valuable clues about the reaction blocked by an antibiotic.

There are two major limitations in the application of this method. In the first place, products of the blocked reaction may not be able to penetrate the cell. For example, borrelidin blocks the conversion of threonine to threonyl-tRNA, yet it is not possible to supply threonyl-tRNA to the cell as a growth factor. Second, reversal of the inhibition may be achieved in other ways than by supplying a product of the blocked reaction. For example, the antagonist may inhibit the entry of the antibiotic into the cell or it may form an inactive complex with the antibiotic.

The search for reversing agents is facilitated by methods that permit screening of many substances with a small amount of effort. A method of this type is the antagonism test, described in Chapter 3 (p. 30). This test was instrumental in the discovery of sideramines, which reverse the inhibition by sideromycins (see p. 94).

As can be seen from the foregoing discussion, the application of the antagonist principle is limited to antibiotics that are antimetabolites, that is, that act at the level of intermediary metabolism on reactions of low-molecular-weight substances. There are many antimetabolites that are not antibiotics, and the development of synthetic antimetabolites played a major role in the history of chemotherapy. On the other hand, many antibiotics are antimetabolites. Some examples were listed in Table 3-1, together with the corresponding metabolites. Besides their production by a living organism there is no inherent difference between naturally occurring antimetabolites and synthetic antimetabolites. Once the chemical structure of an antibiotic is known and reversing agents can be found in cell extracts, the chemical nature of such reversing agents can be surmised from the well-established principle that reversing agents are structurally similar to inhibitors. For example, inhibition by sulfonamides played a major role in the discovery of *p*-aminobenzoic acid, a normal metabolite. In summary, reversal of antibiotic action by a *known* metabolite may localize the site of action of the antibiotic, and reversal by an *unknown* metabolite may give clues as to the chemical nature of the unknown metabolite.

Comparison between Sensitive and Resistant Strains. Mutation to resistance may affect the site of action of an antibiotic, for example, by altering the structure of a sensitive enzyme, and recognition of the alteration may thus uncover the site of action of the antibiotic. For example, mutation to streptomycin resistance causes a change in one of the ribosomal proteins, and it is presumably the function of this protein that is affected by streptomycin in sensitive strains (see p. 105).

Difficulties that may arise in the application of this principle are (1) mutation to resistance may involve functions other than the site of action of the antibiotic, such as permeation of the antibiotic or production of an inactivating enzyme, and (2) a mutation affecting the site of action may also cause other, unrelated changes in cell metabolism.

Mutation to resistance to a given antibiotic often results in cross-resistance to other related antibiotics, and this may be useful in grouping together antibiotics that have a similar mode of action.

Alteration in the Structure of the Antibiotic. Besides the obvious goal of finding more effective antibiotics, the testing of structurally modified compounds permits one to find out which parts of the molecule are necessary for antibiotic activity. Chloramphenicol offers a good example. Structural modification has not resulted in improved activity or better pharmacological properties. However, the following requirements for antibiotic action were discovered.

1. Only the D(–)threo-isomer is active in inhibiting protein synthesis of bacteria.

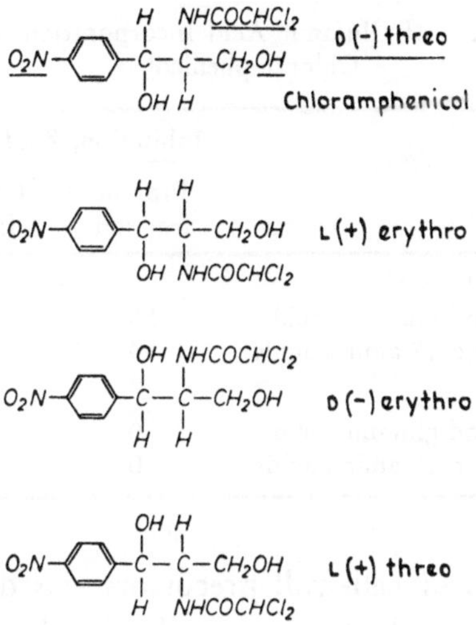

Fig. 5-1. Chloramphenicol and its stereo isomers. Groups essential for chemotherapeutic activity are underlined.

2. The dichloroacetyl moiety can be replaced only by the corresponding bromo-moiety.

3. The terminal primary alcohol group cannot be altered.

4. The benzene ring must carry a substituent group in para position.

Figure 5-1 shows chloramphenicol and its stereo isomers, with the groups required for biological activity underlined.

For studies of this type, chloramphenicol, as well as cycloserine and griseofulvin, are well-suited because they have relatively simple structures and are relatively easy to synthesize. Chloramphenicol inhibits protein synthesis, whereas the L(+)erythro-isomer inhibits the synthesis of D-glutamyl peptides without inhibiting the growth of the bacteria.

This approach has so far not contributed very much to the elucidation of the mode of action of antibiotics.

The Use of Microscopy in the Study of Antibiotic Action. Sublethal doses of antibiotics may lead to morphological changes. For example, in early studies on cell-wall antibiotics (penicillin, bacitracin, cycloserine), the formation of filaments and other bizarre forms suggested a common mode of action of these antibiotics on the cell wall,

Table 5-1   Inhibition of Glutamic Acid Incorporation by Penicillin and
Chloramphenicol

	Inhibition, % of control	
	Protein fraction	Cell-wall fraction
Chloramphenicol		
Glucose and glutamic acid	58	0
Glucose and 18 amino acids	94	0
Penicillin		
Glucose and glutamic acid	0	91
Glucose and 18 amino acids	0	78

before accumulation of cell-wall precursors was demonstrated. Like
cross-resistance, this method may reveal relatedness among different
antibiotics.

Effects on Macromolecular Incorporation. As an example of this
technique, Table 5-1 shows the effects of penicillin and chloramphenicol on the incorporation of glutamic acid into proteins and cell-wall
constituents. The data by themselves tell us little more than to say
that the two antibiotics have different modes of action. In conjunction
with other information, however, they do substantiate the conclusion
that penicillin inhibits cell-wall synthesis without affecting protein
synthesis, whereas chloramphenicol inhibits protein synthesis without
affecting cell-wall synthesis.

Antibiotics Affecting Cell-Wall Formation

By means of mechanical disintegration and fractionation followed
by chemical analysis and electron microscopy, the bacterial cell wall
has been shown to consist of several layers. In gram-positive bacteria
the wall structure is relatively simple. The main layer is the peptidoglycan layer, which in many species is surrounded by a teichoic acid
layer. In some species there is a layer of polysaccharide. In gram-
negative bacteria the wall is more complex, consisting of a peptidoglycan layer surrounded by layers of lipoproteins and lipopoly-
saccharides. In both gram-positive and gram-negative bacteria the
wall surrounds the cytoplasmic membrane and lends rigid support to
an otherwise fragile cell.

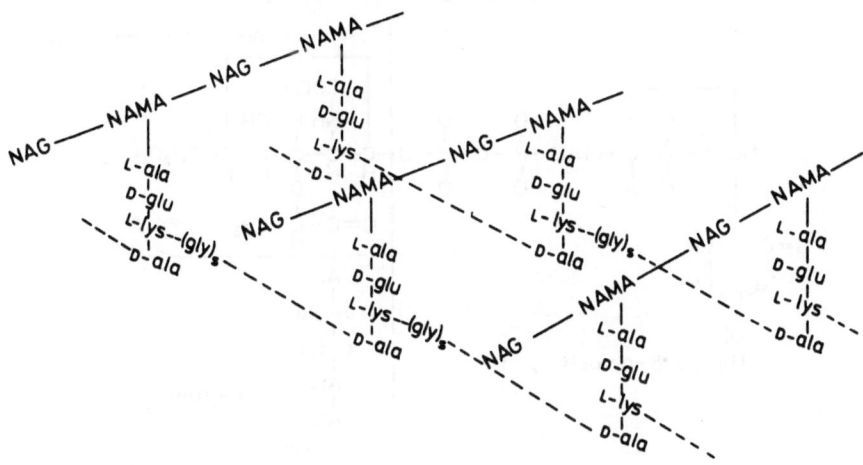

Fig. 5-2. Structure of peptidoglycan of *S. aureus* showing interpeptide bridges composed of glycine subunits. (From Mandelstam, J. and K. McQuillen, ed., *Biochemistry of Bacterial Growth*, Wiley, New York, 1968)

Of primary interest in the present context is the peptidoglycan layer, because all known cell-wall antibiotics act on the formation of this part of the wall. As there is no comparable structure in animal cells, specific action on this layer ensures selective toxicity against bacteria.

The peptidoglycan layer is a giant polymeric network enclosing the whole cell like a corset. Its structure is indicated schematically in Fig. 5-2. It has the following general features, with variations and additions being present in different groups of bacteria.

1. Alternating units of N-acetyl-D-glucosamine and N-acetylmuramic acid are in β-1,4 linkage.

2. A tetrapeptide is attached to muramic acid and contains the sequence, starting from the amino terminal end, L-alanine-γ-D-isoglutamine-L-lysine-D-alanine. L-Lysine may be replaced by other diamino acids, such as *meso*-diaminopimelic acid (*meso*-DAP), LL-DAP, ornithine, or α,γ-diaminobutyric acid.

3. The tetrapeptide chains are at least partially cross-linked to each other, the COOH group of D-alanine in one chain being linked to the NH$_2$ group of lysine (or its substitute) in a second chain. This linkage may be either direct (in *E. coli*) or via an oligopeptide bridge (in *S. aureus*). The degree of cross-linking varies from one organism to another and also from one stage of the growth cycle to another.

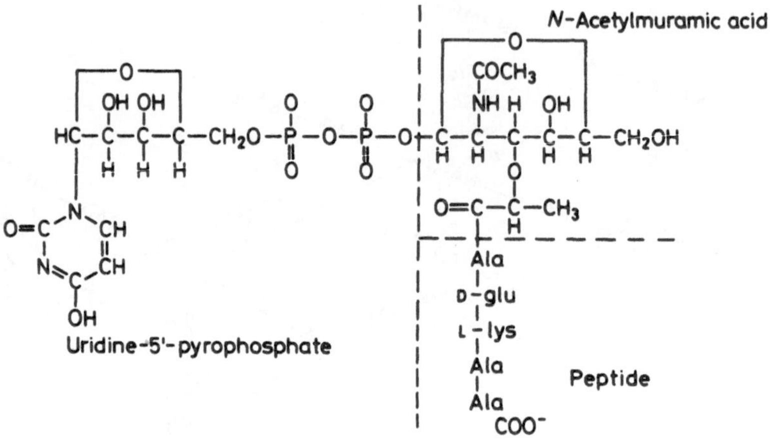

Fig. 5-3. Structure of the major UDP-acetylmuramyl-peptide accumulating in a penicillin-treated culture of *S. aureus*. (From J. T. Park in S. T. Cowan and E. Rowalf, eds., *The Strategy of Chemotherapy*. Eighth Symposium of the Society for General Microbiology. Cambridge University Press, 1958.)

As the cell grows, new wall is laid down; this is achieved through the action of hydrolases, which open up parts of the peptidoglycan, and synthetases (see below), which add on new units into the network. To maintain normal growth the actions of these two types of enzymes must be balanced against each other. If the synthetases are inhibited, excessive hydrolysis will occur, which may lead to cell death since the weakened supporting structure would not be able to withstand the high intracellular osmotic pressure and the cell lyses. The following antibiotics interfere with peptidoglycan synthesis: penicillins, cephalosporins, vancomycin, ristocetin, bacitracin, D-cycloserine, O-carbamyl-D-serine, enduracidin, prasinomycins, and phosphoromycin.

As early as 1949, J. T. Park and coworkers demonstrated that in the presence of sublethal concentrations of penicillin, *S. aureus* accumulates a then-unknown family of compounds ("Park compounds"). Later the structure shown in Fig. 5-3 was assigned to the main member of this group. The right-hand side of this structure is identical with the muramyl peptide portion of the peptidoglycan (Fig. 5-2) except for the extra D-alanine unit.

The biosynthesis of the peptidoglycan takes place in distinct stages, each of which occurs at a different site in the cell.

Stage 1. Assembly of the building blocks. The uridine nucleotide precursors of N-acetylglucosamine (GlcNAc) and the muramyl-peptide are synthesized in the cytoplasm. This process is shown in Fig. 5-4. D-cycloserine and O-carbamyl-D-serine inhibit the racemization of L-alanine and the formation of the D-ala-D-ala dipeptide. The inhibition can be reversed by D-alanine. Recently a new antibiotic, phosphonomycin, has been shown to block the formation of muramic acid by inhibiting the condensation of phosphoenol pyruvate and N-acetylglucosamine.

Stage 2. Transfer of the nucleotide precursors to the growing peptidoglycan chain. The muramyl peptide and acetyl-glucosamine portions of the nucleotides are first transferred to a membrane-bound phospholipid carrier (identified as a C_{55}-polyisoprenoid alcohol phosphate), giving rise to a disaccharide-pentapeptide-P-P-phospholipid (see Fig. 5-5). At this point further modifications may occur on the peptide chain (for example, in *S. aureus* addition of a pentaglycine residue to L-lysine via glycyl-tRNA and an amide group to the α-carboxyl group of glutamic acid) leading to the finished peptidoglycan subunit. The latter is transferred to the acceptor end of a peptidoglycan chain, and the P-P-phospholipid is released. This transfer is inhibited by vancomycin and ristocetin. Next, one phosphate is split off from the P-P-phospholipid. The latter then is ready to reenter the cycle. The dephosphorylation is blocked by bacitracin.

Stage 3. Cross-linking between linear peptidoglycan strands. This reaction occurs on the outside of the cell membrane. It involves a transpeptidation between two peptide moieties with the elimination of D-alanine (Fig. 5-6). This is the reaction that is sensitive to penicillins and cephalosporins. It has been suggested by Strominger that because of structural similarity penicillin acts as an antagonist of the acyl-D-alanyl-D-alanine peptide in the enzymatic transpeptidation.

It should be noted that an understanding of the overall process of peptidoglycan synthesis helps to elucidate the mode of action of cell-wall antibiotics, and further, that the availability of these antibiotics has been instrumental in working out the steps in peptidoglycan synthesis.

With the available description of the mode of action of penicillin it is possible to explain several previously observed phenomena elicited by penicillin.

1. Penicillin requires growth of cells in order to kill them; the faster the growth, the more effective is its action.

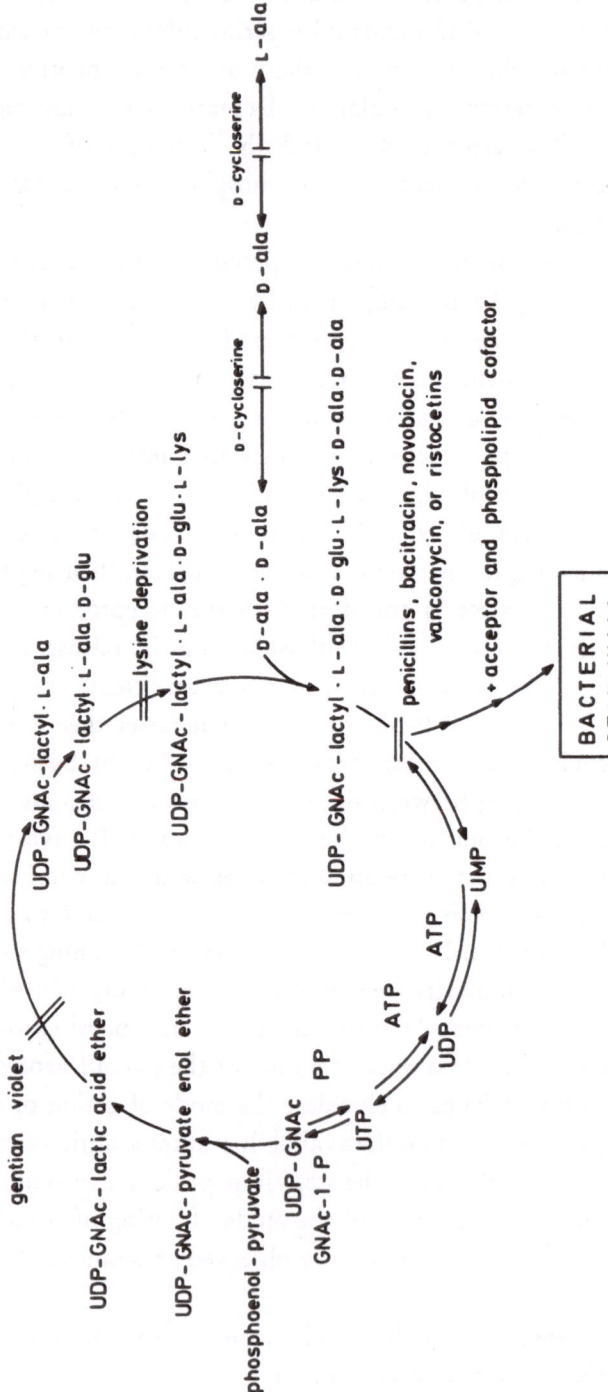

Fig. 5-4. Biosynthesis of the uridine nucleotide precursors of the peptidoglycan. The points of inhibition by various substances are indicated. (From J. L. Strominger in Bücher, Th. and H. Sies, eds., *Inhibitors Tools in Cell Research*, Springer-Verlag, New York, 1969.)

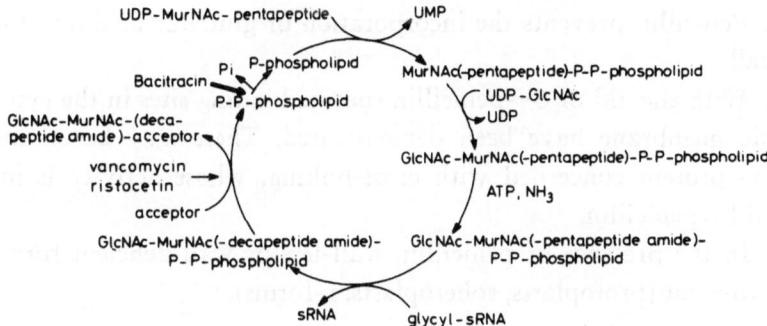

Fig. 5-5. Phospholipid cycle in peptidoglycan synthesis in *S. aureus*. The reactions in which the lipid intermediates are modified are included in this cycle. (See Bücher and Sies.)

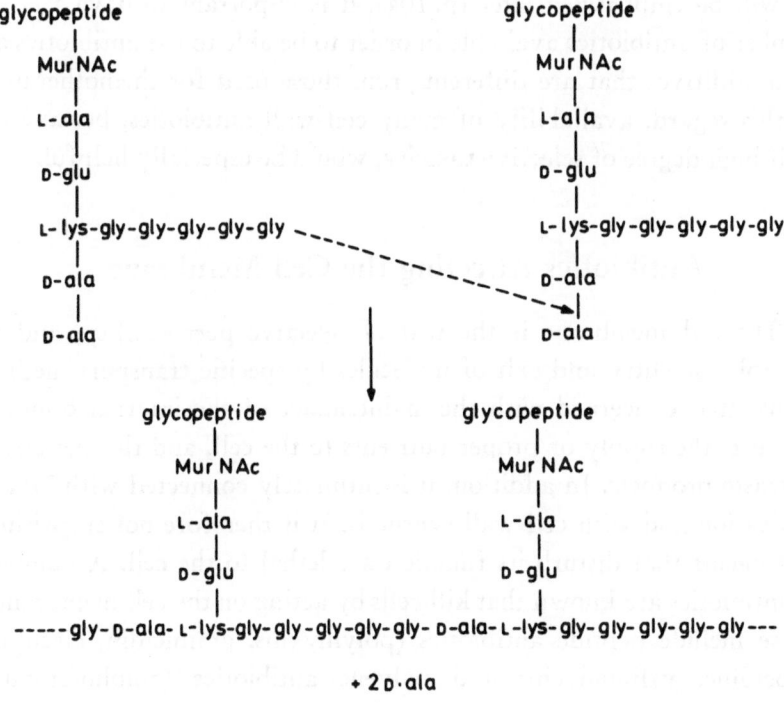

Fig. 5-6. Transpeptidation of two linear peptidoglycan strands with closure of the interpeptide bridges and elimination of D-alanine. (See Bücher and Sies.)

2. Penicillin prevents the incorporation of glutamic acid into the cell wall.

3. With the aid of S^{35}-penicillin specific binding sites in the cytoplasmic membrane have been demonstrated. These may be on the enzyme protein concerned with cross-linking, whose activity is inhibited by penicillin.

4. In the presence of penicillin, wall-less or wall-deficient forms may grow out (protoplasts, spheroplasts, L-forms).

Two other cell-wall antibiotics have been mentioned, enduracidin and prasinomycin. In the presence of these substances muramyl peptides accumulate, but the precise mode of action has not yet been determined. Besides being possibly useful for chemotherapy, these antibiotics may turn out to be effective as additives in animal feeds. As will be emphasized later (p. 104), it is important to have a large number of antibiotics available in order to be able to use antibiotics as food additives that are different from those used for chemotherapy. In this regard, availability of many cell-wall antibiotics, because of their high degree of selective toxicity, would be especially helpful.

Antibiotics Affecting the Cell Membrane

The cell membrane is the seat of selective permeability, and it controls the entry and exit of molecules by specific transport mechanisms. It is concerned with the maintenance of the internal osmotic pressure, the supply of proper nutrients to the cell, and the excretion of waste products. In addition, it is intimately connected with DNA replication and with cell-wall synthesis. It is therefore not surprising that agents that disturb its function are lethal to the cell. A number of antibiotics are known that kill cells by acting on the cell membrane. These include peptide antibiotics (polymyxins, gramicidin, circulin, tyrocidine, valinomycin) and polyene antibiotics (amphotericins, nystatin, filipin, candicin). As might be expected from the presence of similar membranes in all organisms, these antibiotics do not exhibit the same degree of selective toxicity as the cell-wall antibiotics. In medicine most of them are too toxic for systemic use, but they can be used topically.

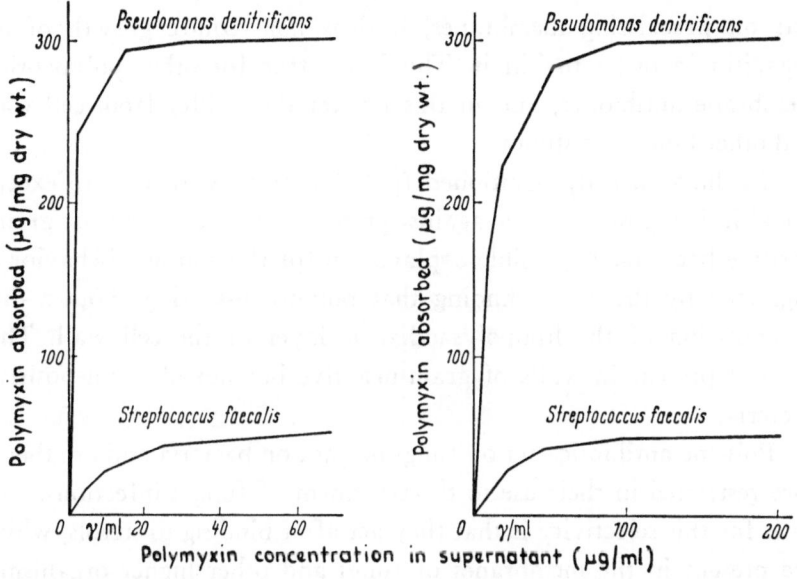

Fig. 5-7. Absorption of polymyxin by sensitive and resistant bacteria. Left: whole cells; right: cell-wall preparation. (Modified from B. A. Newton in Cowan and Rowatt, eds., *The Strategy of Chemotherapy* Cambridge University Press, 1958.)

In the case of polymyxin, action on the membrane was suggested in experiments performed by Newton, who demonstrated binding of the antibiotic to the cytoplasmic membrane. Data on binding to whole cells and a cell-wall fraction (presumably containing membrane material) are shown in Fig. 5-7. A marked difference is found between a sensitive *(P. denitrificans)* and a resistant *(S. faecalis)* organism, whether one uses whole cells or the cell-wall fraction. Another approach used by Newton utilized a fluorescent derivative of polymyxin. This material was found to accumulate only on the surface of bacteria. It also was shown that it binds to extracted phospholipids, and there was more binding to phospholipids extracted from sensitive bacteria than to phospholipids extracted from resistant bacteria.

The damage caused by polymyxin to the cell membrane can be recognized in several ways: leakage of soluble constituents (various metabolites, including nucleotides), penetration of normally excluded substances into the cell, and fluorescent staining by a dye that fluoresces only after being bound to protein and that does not stain cells that have not been exposed to polymyxin. Because polymyxin acts on preexisting membranes, it does not require growth of an organism in order to kill it. This holds true for other polypeptide membrane antibiotics, and in this respect they differ from cell-wall and other kinds of antibiotics.

We have already mentioned (p. 10) that polymyxins are exceptional in being more active against gram-negative than against gram-positive bacteria. A possible explanation for this unusual behavior is suggested by the recent finding that polymyxins bring about a disorganization of the lipopolysaccharide layer of the cell wall. This layer is present in walls of gram-negative but not of gram-positive bacteria.

Polyene antibiotics act on fungi but not on bacteria and are therefore restricted in their use to the treatment of fungal infections. The basis for this selectivity is that they act after binding to sterols, which are present in the membranes of fungi and other higher organisms, but not in bacterial membranes. Polyenes can cause hemolysis *in vitro*, presumably because red-blood-cell membranes contain sterols. The polyene amphotericin B can be used in the treatment of systemic infections, but a frequently encountered side effect is hemolytic anemia.

In connection with membrane function a type of antibiotic may be mentioned here that is of interest to basic bacterial biochemistry and physiology but has so far not been therapeutically useful. These antibiotics are concerned with the transport of alkali-metal ions across cytoplasmic membranes and mitochondrial membranes. Two groups of substances fall into this category, the first consisting of neutral polypeptides or polyesters containing a large ring structure, the second consisting of a large carboxylic acid containing many rings with oxygens inserted in ether linkage. Examples of both groups are shown in Fig. 5-8.

In the first group are included valinomycin (I), the macrotetrolides (nonactin (II), monactin, dinactin, trinactin) and the enniatins. These molecules can form complexes with alkali-metal ions. The complexes have a spherical shape, with the metal ion being in the center of the sphere. The many oxygen atoms of the molecule are directed toward the center of the sphere, whereas the lipophilic groups are directed toward the outside. Complexes formed with potassium ions are more stable than complexes formed with sodium ions. It has been demon-

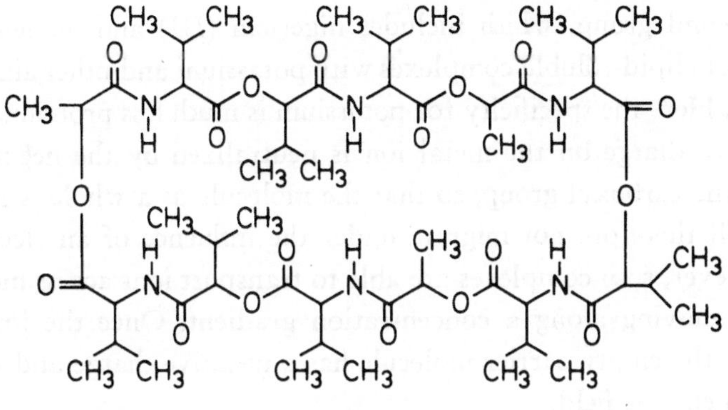

Fig. 5-8. Examples of ion-selective antibiotics. I = valinomycin; II = nonactin; III = nigericin.

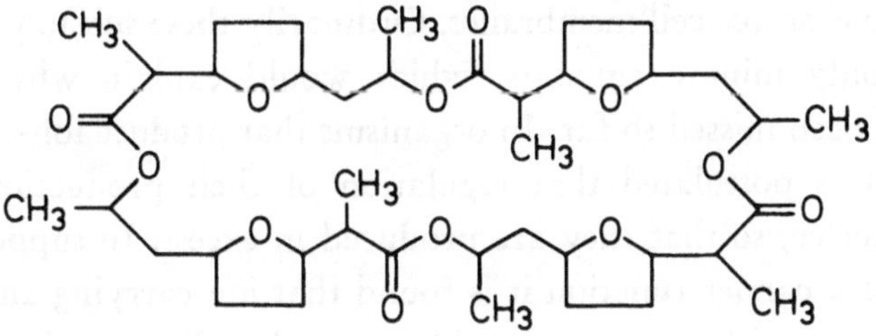

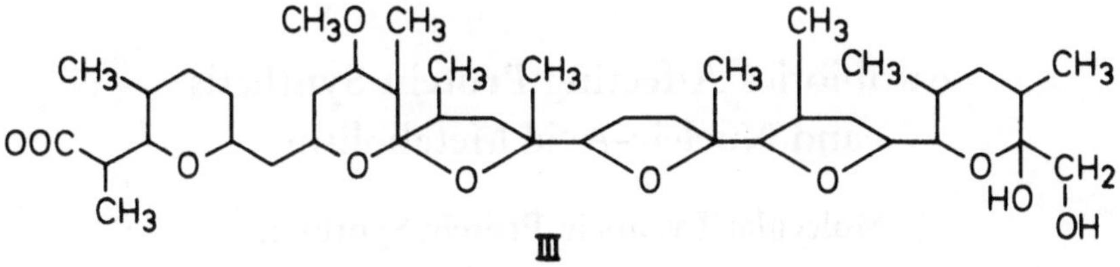

strated that these complexes, being positively charged, will migrate across artificial membranes under the influence of an electric field. Such a carrier mechanism can go far to explain the effects that have been produced by these antibiotics in whole cells of bacteria and in mitochondria.

The second group, which includes nigericin (III) and monensin, can also form lipid-soluble complexes with potassium and other alkali-metal ions. Here the specificity for potassium is much less pronounced. The positive charge on the metal ion is neutralized by the negative charge of the carboxyl group, so that the molecule as a whole is neutral. It will therefore not migrate under the influence of an electric field. However, such complexes are able to transport ions across membranes by moving along a concentration gradient. Once the ion is discharged, the empty carrier molecule has a negative charge and will move in an electric field.

The existence of these ion-carrying antibiotics opens up the possibility that such molecules may exist in many types of cells as normal carriers of ions across cell membranes. Ordinarily these substances are present in only minute amounts, which would explain why their presence has been missed so far. In organisms that produce ion-carrier antibiotics it is postulated that regulation of their production has become defective, so that they are produced in excess. In support of the notion of a carrier function it is found that ion-carrying antibiotics belonging to either group are able to bind to lipoproteins. If it turns out that these substances do have a general ion-carrier function, they would presumably be produced during growth of the cells and would thus be primary metabolites rather than secondary metabolites.

Antibiotics Affecting Protein Synthesis and Nucleic-Acid Metabolism

Molecular Events in Protein Synthesis

The unraveling of the mechanism of protein synthesis is at the center of the field of molecular biology. The flow of information from DNA to RNA to protein is known as the "central dogma." The details are described in many places, including most of the recent textbooks of biochemistry, microbiology, and genetics. Here we confine ourselves to a brief account, sufficient to give a background for a discussion of antibiotics affecting nucleic acid and protein synthesis. For more extensive treatments, references are listed at the end of the chapter.

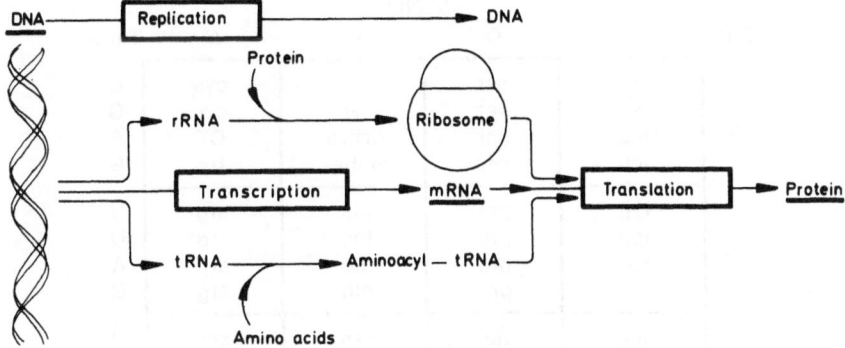

Fig. 5-9. Diagram showing the DNA-coded activities: replication, transcription, and translation.

The events of protein synthesis and processes associated with it are presented schematically in Fig. 5-9. The first event is a transcription of one of the strands of the double-stranded DNA molecule to form a messenger RNA (mRNA) molecule. This reaction is carried out by a complex enzyme, DNA-dependent, RNA polymerase. The mRNA molecule is then translated into a protein molecule. This involves attachment of a ribosome at one end of the mRNA molecule and movement of the ribosome along the mRNA to the other end. As the ribosome moves along, it assembles amino acids into a peptide chain. When all the amino acids of a protein have been assembled, the completed peptide chain is released from the ribosome-mRNA complex. Several ribosomes may travel along one mRNA molecule at the same time, generating several polypeptide chains simultaneously. A complex consisting of one mRNA molecule attached to several ribosomes is called a polysome. In bacteria, translation starts as soon as the mRNA begins to be released from the DNA template, so that transcription and translation occur simultaneously and in the same location. We shall return to a more detailed acount of translation after we have considered some genetic aspects of protein synthesis.

The genetic information is encoded in the sequence of nucleic acid bases of the DNA double helix. The remarkable property of specific base pairing permits the DNA strands to act as templates in the synthesis of new nucleic-acid molecules. Adenine always pairs with thymine (or uracil for RNA synthesis), guanine with cytosine. The

| First | Second | | | | Third |
	U	C	A	G	
U	phe	ser	tyr	cys	U
	phe	ser	tyr	cys	C
	leu	ser	ochre	CT	A
	leu	ser	amber	try	G
C	leu	pro	his	arg	U
	leu	pro	his	arg	C
	leu	pro	gln	arg	A
	leu	pro	gln	arg	G
A	ile	thr	asn	ser	U
	ile	thr	asn	ser	C
	ile	thr	lys	arg	A
	met, fmet	thr	lys	arg	G
G	val	ala	asp	gly	U
	val	ala	asp	gly	C
	val	ala	glu	gly	A
	val	ala	glu	gly	G

Fig. 5-10. The genetic code. (From Lewin, B. M., *The Molecular Basis of Gene Expression*, Wiley-Interscience, London, 1970.)

new strand of nucleic acid made is thus complementary to the strand that served as its template. On the next round of synthesis, the new strand gives rise to a sequence that is exactly like the one from which it was derived. A strand of DNA is thus able to reproduce itself via the intermediary formation of a complementary strand. During transcription the mRNA formed is complementary to the DNA strand that served as its template and has the same sequence as the second DNA strand of the double helix.

The unit of transcription, that is, the length of DNA that is transcribed into one piece of mRNA, is called an operon. It is a long stretch of DNA (several thousand nucleotide pairs) and consists of either one or several cistrons (genes). A segment at one end of an operon, called the promoter, is the site at which RNA polymerase attaches and begins transcription.

Translation depends on the recognition of three consecutive nucleotides as a signal to insert an amino acid. Each amino acid is determined by a different triplet of nucleotides (codon), but there may be several codons for a given amino acid. The array of possible triplets, called the genetic code, is shown in Fig. 5-10. Translation, in the final analysis, also depends on base pairing. As we shall see shortly, it is the pairing of three nucleotides in a codon with three corresponding bases in the anticodon site of a transfer RNA (tRNA) molecule that determines which amino acid is going to be inserted into the growing peptide chain.

The unit of translation is the cistron, and it codes in most cases for a single complete polypeptide chain. When a ribosome has reached the end of a cistron, it encounters a chain-terminating codon that is responsible for the release of the completed polypeptide chain from the ribosome.

It should be noted that mRNA is not the only kind of RNA transcribed from DNA. We have already mentioned tRNA. In addition there is ribosomal RNA (rRNA), which makes up a large part of the ribosome. Neither tRNA nor rRNA is translated into protein. The relationship of transcription to translation, the replication of DNA, and the formation of tRNA and rRNA and their relationship to protein synthesis are all shown in Fig. 5-9.

We shall now consider the translation process in somewhat greater detail. The process can be subdivided into three phases: (I) formation of an initiation complex, (II) chain elongation, and (III) chain termination. Phase I involves the binding of the first amino acid, linked to a species of tRNA, to one of the two subunits of the ribosome. In bacteria the first amino acid is always methionine, and its amino group is formylated after attachment to transfer RNA to give a molecule of formylmethionyl-tRNA (f-met-tRNA) .The two bacterial ribosomal subunits have sedimentation constants of 30s and 50s, and f-met-tRNA attaches to the 30s subunit. The complete ribosome has a sedimentation constant of 70s. Before going any further with the discussion of phase I, we should say a word about the formation of the aminoacyl-tRNA compound.

For each amino acid there is an activating enzyme, which catalyzes the coupling of the amino acid to the corresponding tRNA, with the utilization of ATP as energy source. There may be one or several species of tRNA for a given amino acid. Activating enzymes are very specific and do not place amino acids onto the wrong king of tRNA. Formation of the aminoacyl-tRNA compound passes through an intermediary aminoacyl-AMP-enzyme complex. Thus the formation of methionyl-tRNA may be written as follows:

$$\text{ATP} + \text{methionine} + \text{enzyme} \xrightarrow{\text{Mg}^{2+}} \text{enzyme-methionine-AMP} + \text{PP}_i$$

$$\text{enzyme-methionine-AMP} + \text{tRNA} \rightarrow \text{met-tRNA} + \text{enzyme} + \text{AMP}.$$

A specific formylase catalyzes the reaction:

$$\text{met-tRNA} + \text{formyltetrahydrofolate} \rightarrow \text{N-formyl-met-tRNA}.$$

To continue with phase I, f-met-tRNA forms a complex with a 30s subunit attached to an mRNA molecule. Three initiation factors and GTP are required for this process. A 50s ribosomal subunit is added on, and the complex is then ready to receive a second aminoacyl-tRNA and to start polypeptide chain formation. The steps involved in the formation of the complex are shown schematically in Fig. 5-11. Note that the initiator codon is AUG and that the attachment of f-met-tRNA occurs on a specific site of the ribosome, called the A site, followed by movement to the P site.

Phase II (see Fig. 5-12) begins when a second aminoacyl-tRNA has been placed into the A site, with its anticodon (in this case CGG) paired with the second codon (GCC). Binding of the second aminoacyl-tRNA requires GTP and the presence of two binding factors. A peptide bond is formed between the carboxyl group of f-met-tRNA and the amino group of the incoming amino acid. This reaction is catalyzed by a ribosome-bound peptidyl transferase. The tRNA portion of f-met-tRNA is released, and a dipeptide is now attached to the tRNA of the second amino acid. This peptidyl-tRNA moves over to the P site, liberating the A site for the next addition. This translocation reaction requires GTP and a translocation factor, G. Note that in this translocation mRNA also shifts position so that at the end of the process the next codon in line is below the empty A site.

Phase III occurs when the codon below the empty A site is a chain-terminating codon, for example UAA. There is no tRNA with the corresponding anticodon, and therefore no amino acid can be inserted. Instead the peptide chain is split off from the tRNA, and the tRNA is released from the ribosome. The process of chain termination also requires the presence of several protein-termination factors. The 70s ribosomes eventually dissociate into 30s and 50s subunits, and this

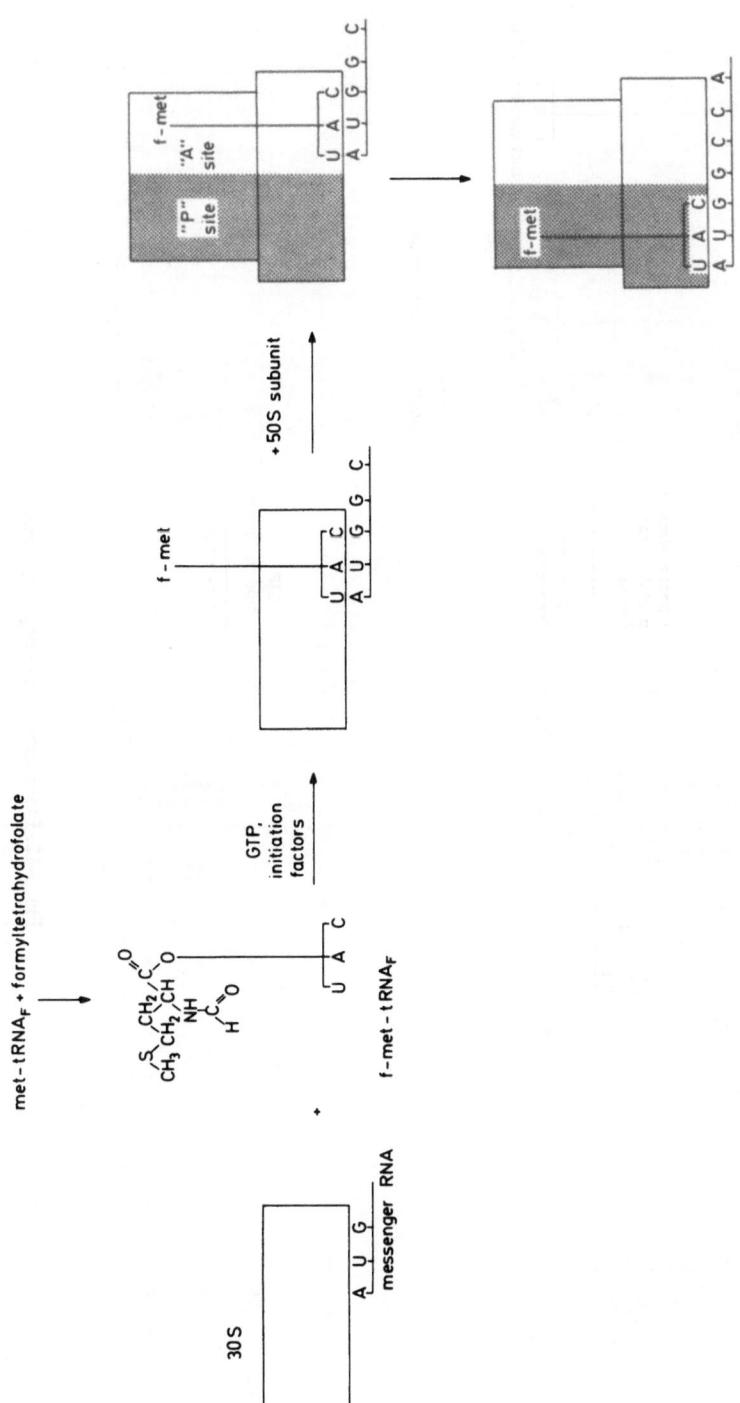

Fig. 5-11. Formation of the initiation complex.

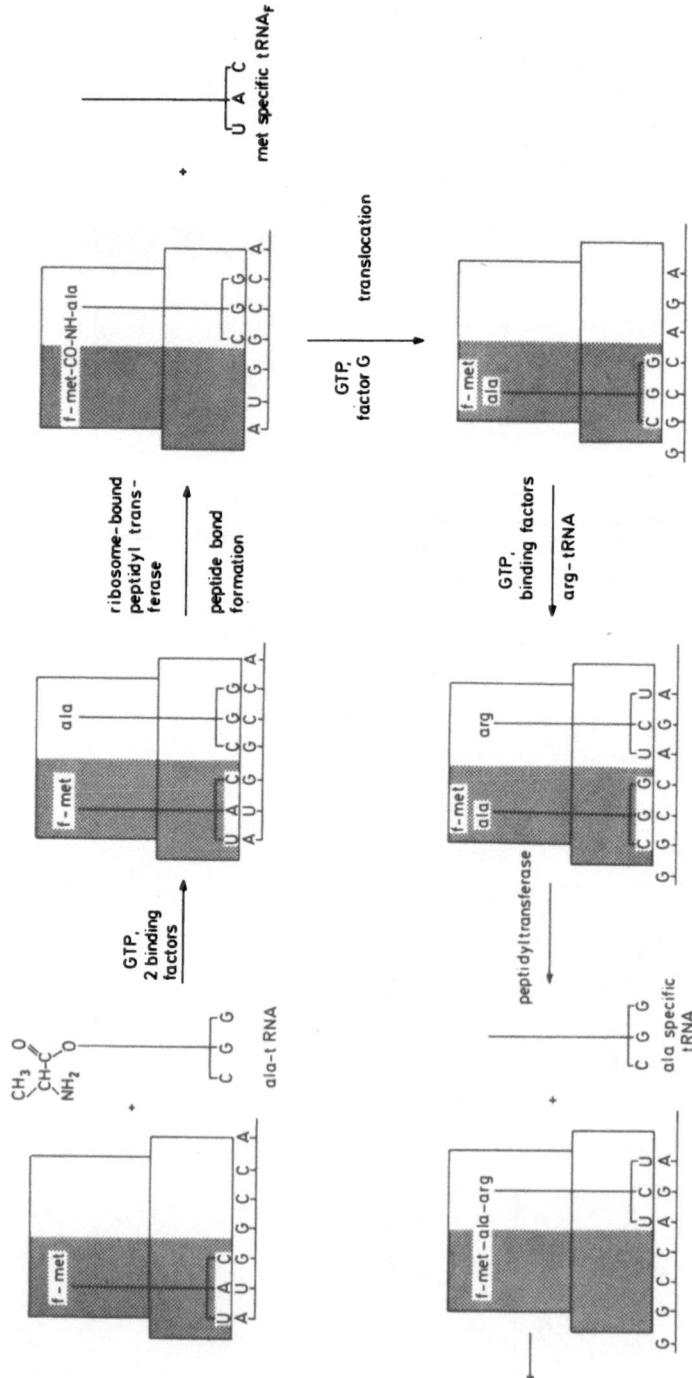

Fig. 5-12. Elongation of the peptide chain.

requires reaction with a dissociation factor before a new initiation complex can be formed.

Antibiotics Inhibiting the Synthesis of Nucleic Acids and Proteins

As indicated by the arrows in Fig. 5-9, we can denote four sites of action for antibiotics that inhibit the synthesis of nucleic acids and proteins: (1) replication of DNA; (2) transcription; (3) formation of aminoacyl-tRNAs; and (4) translation. Table 5-2 lists some of

Table 5-2   Antibiotics Interfering with the Synthesis of Nucleic Acids and Proteins

1 DNA replication	2 Transcription	1 and 2	3 Aminoacyl- tRNA formation	4 Translation
Phleomycin	Actinomycins	Anthracyclines	Borrelidin	Chloramphenicol
Bleomycin	Chromomycins			Puromycin
Edeine	Echinomycin			Gougerotin
Mitomycins	Rifamycins			Streptomycin
Porfiromycins	Cordycepin			Neomycin
	Streptolydigin			Kanamycin
				Paromomycin
				Streptogramins
				Macrolide group
				Carbomycin
				Erythromycin
				Lankamycin
				Methymycin
				Spectinomycins
				Thiostrepton
				group
				Lincomycins
				Sparsomycin
				Cycloheximide
				Fusidic Acid
				Tetracyclines

the antibiotics interfering with each of these processes. We shall first discuss antibiotics that inhibit nucleic acid synthesis. As might be expected, a drug that binds to DNA interferes with both DNA replication and RNA synthesis. In some cases the effect is much stronger on one of these processes than on the other, and such agents can be listed under only one category (either 1 or 2). In other cases both processes are affected more or less equally, and such agents are listed under both categories (1 and 2). However, drugs that act specifically on the enzymes of DNA replication or on RNA polymerase are found to affect, respectively, only DNA replication or only RNA synthesis.

Antibiotics affecting nucleic-acid synthesis are in general not selectively toxic against bacteria and are therefore not useful chemotherapeutic agents. They have been valuable as tools in biochemical studies of nucleic acid metabolism. Some of them have been classified as antitumor agents and have shown promise in the treatment of cancer.

DNA Replication

Phleomycin and *bleomycin* are copper-containing antibiotic complexes obtained from a species of *Streptomyces* and are effective against a variety of bacteria. Bleomycin is used in cancer therapy. Evidence has been obtained that these complexes bind to DNA. Phleomycin inhibits DNA polymerase I in extracts, but much higher concentrations are required than to inhibit DNA synthesis in whole cells of *E. coli.* This is of interest in regard to recent findings, which suggest that DNA replication may not be mediated by DNA polymerase I. *Edeine* is a basic polypeptide produced by *Bacillus brevis.* It inhibits DNA synthesis of bacteria at concentrations at which protein and RNA synthesis are not affected. The *mitomycins* and *porfiromycins*, produced by several species of *Streptomyces*, are inactive by themselves, but are reduced inside the cell to active derivatives. They form cross-links between complementary DNA strands and also act as alkylating agents of DNA. The latter activity confers on these compounds the ability to produce mutations. However, the actual killing may not be caused by either activity. Besides the effect on DNA replication, a number of secondary effects have been observed, including DNA breakdown, inhibition of RNA synthesis, and inhibition of induced-enzyme formation.

Transcription

Of the antibiotics affecting transcription, the most thoroughly studied are the *actinomycins*. Actinomycin D is a bright-red polypeptide compound in which two peptide chains are attached to a

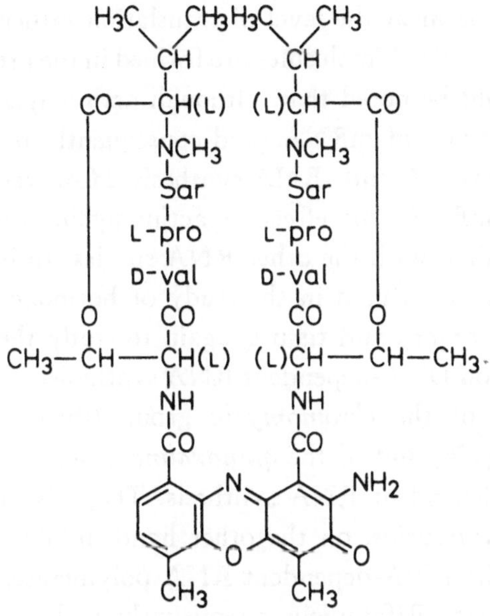

Fig. 5-13. Structure of actinomycin D. (From Gottlieb and Shaw, see References, All Aspects, no. 2.)

chromophoric ring system (Fig. 5-13). Actinomycins form stable complexes with double-stranded but not single-stranded DNA. The degree of binding depends on the guanine content of the DNA. Presumably the drug is located in the minor groove of the DNA helix and is held in place by hydrogen bonds to guanylic-acid residues. Binding of actinomycin to DNA can be detected by a change in its absorption spectrum.

Exposure of sensitive cells to actinomycin results in immediate cessation of DNA-dependent RNA synthesis. With much higher concentrations DNA synthesis is also arrested. Because of its specific action, actinomycin D does not inhibit replication of single-stranded RNA viruses and phages. However, replication of double-stranded RNA viruses is inhibited.

Actinomycin D has been an important tool in the study of macromolecular metabolism. It has been used to differentiate those processes that depend on DNA-mediated RNA synthesis from others that do not. For example, if it can be shown that formation of an enzyme is induced in the presence of actinomycin, induction of enzyme synthesis can be said to occur at the level of translation rather than transcription, as no new mRNA molecules are formed in the presence of actinomycin. It should be noted that, although actinomycin has been used mainly in the study of mRNA (and consequently protein) synthesis, it also inhibits tRNA and rRNA synthesis. However, because of the instability of mRNA, the effect of actinomycin is more immediate and dramatic than with the other RNA species. In higher organisms actinomycin has been used in the study of hormone action and differentiation of organs and tissues, again to study the dependence of various phases on DNA-dependent RNA synthesis.

Antibiotics of the *chromomycin* group (chromomycin, mithramycin, olivomycin) and of the *quinoxaline* group (echinomycin) also inhibit DNA-dependent RNA synthesis. They also form complexes with DNA. *Rifamycins*, on the other hand, inhibit RNA synthesis by acting on the DNA-dependent RNA polymerase, rather than on the DNA template. Rifampicin, a semisynthetic derivative of rifamycin, has been shown to bind to the free enzyme. It inhibits initiation of transcription but not the completion of RNA chain synthesis started before addition of the drug. Its effect on RNA synthesis, unlike that of actinomycin, is therefore not immediate. Rifampicin-resistant mutants of *E. coli* have been isolated in which the RNA polymerase is altered and no longer binds rifampicin.

Antibiotics Acting on DNA Replication and Transcription

The *anthracycline* antibiotics (daunomycin, cinerubin, nogalamycin) affect both DNA replication and DNA transcription. Thus they block the template activity of DNA for both processes. These substances form complexes with DNA.

Formation of Aminoacyl-tRNAs

Only one antibiotic has been found which acts at this level, *borrelidin*. This substance inhibits specifically the activity of the threonine-activating enzyme, thus preventing the formation of threonyl-tRNA. The specific action of borrelidin makes it a valuable tool for biochemical investigations, and it has been used to study the role of threonyl-tRNA in repression of the enzymes involved in threonine biosynthesis.

Translation

The majority of the antibiotics affecting nucleic acid and protein synthesis act at the level of translation. Chemically they form a very heterogeneous group. Among them are many therapeutically useful compounds. This attests to one or more differences in the mechanism of translation between bacteria (prokaryotes) and cells of higher forms (eukaryotes), which permits them to exhibit selective toxicity. One difference is in the structure of ribosomes. Bacterial ribosomes have a sedimentation value of 70s and are composed of 30s and 50s subunits. Mammalian ribosomes have a sedimentation value of 80s and are composed of 40s and 60s subunits. It should be pointed out that ribosomes of mitochondria and chloroplasts resemble bacterial ribosomes, and as a consequence protein synthesis in these organelles has a sensitivity spectrum similar to that of bacteria. Mitochondria also have circular DNA, like bacteria.

Table 5-3 summarizes information about the mode of action of the principal antibiotics affecting translation. We shall discuss a few of

Table 5-3   Action of Antibiotics Affecting Translation

Antibiotic	Subunit affected	Probable mode of action
Streptomycin	30 S	Distorts configuration of 30 S subunit. Inhibits initiation?
Tetracyclines	30 S	Blocks binding of aminoacyl-tRNA.
Puromycin	50 S	An analog of aminoacyl-tRNA, clears P site of peptidyl-tRNA.
Chloramphenicol	50 S	Inhibits peptidyl transferase.
Fusidic acid	50 S	Blocks G-factor activity.

these agents in detail. The chief methods used to obtain this information were: (1) binding of radioactive antibiotics to ribosomes or competition with such binding; (2) reconstitution of hybrid ribosomes from ribosome subunits derived from antibiotic-sensitive and anti-biotic-resistant cells, followed by studies on sensitivity of the recon-stituted ribosomes to the corresponding antibiotic; and (3) effects of antibiotics on a function specifically associated with one subunit and amenable to study in the absence of the other subunit.

Puromycin. It is advantageous to start with this antibiotic, because it has a clear-cut mode of action and can be used as a tool to determine the mode of action of other antibiotics. It acts as a chain terminator during elongation of growing peptide chains and causes their release from the ribosome. It can be considered as a structural analog of an aminoacyl-tRNA (see Fig. 4-13), and it will form a peptide bond with the peptidyl-tRNA located in the P site of the ribosome. As it does not have enough affinity for the ribosome to retain anchorage, the puromycin-peptide chain comes off the ribosome. If a second antibiotic prevents chain release by puromycin in an *in vitro* system, it can be said to exert its effect prior to the stage at which puromycin acts (for example, chloramphenicol, sparsomycin, erythromycin, fusidic acid).

Puromycin inhibits protein synthesis in all types of cells and is therefore not useful for therapy of infectious diseases. Another antibiotic, *gougerotin,* is structurally similar to puromycin, except that it contains a pyrimidine instead of a purine ring (Fig. 4-14). This substance does not form a peptide bond with the last amino acid of the growing peptide chain, but acts as a competitive inhibitor of aminoacyl-tRNA or puromycin in peptide-bond synthesis. Thus it also prevents elongation of peptide chains but does not cause their release from the ribosome.

Chloramphenicol. This antibiotic has been used a great deal in studies in which it was necessary to specifically inhibit protein synthesis without interfering with other macromolecular synthesis. For example, the conclusion that incorporation of an amino acid into the cell wall involves processes that are different from incorporation into protein (see p. 68) is based on the finding that the latter, not the former, process can be inhibited by chloramphenicol. Inhibition by chloramphenicol is reversible, and the drug is bacteristatic. It binds to 50s subunits and seems to interfere with the peptidyl transferase reaction. As would be expected, in an *in vitro* system is prevents chain release by puromycin.

A number of other antibiotics (macrolides, lincomycin, celesticetin) interfere competitively with the binding of ^{14}C-chloramphenicol to 50s subunits, and this has provided evidence for the conclusion that these antibiotics also bind to 50s subunits. Chloramphenicol does not bind to the 80s ribosomes of higher forms, and this is presumably the basis for its selective toxicity. It does bind to mitochondrial ribosomes and chloroplast ribosomes.

In the presence of chloramphenicol bacteria are not able to carry ribosome synthesis to completion; instead they accumulate unfinished ribosomal precursor particles, which have been characterized. Chloramphenicol is thus of value in studying the synthesis and assembly of ribosomes.

Streptomycin. This (Fig. 6-7) is the most widely studied of the antibiotics that act on 30s subunits. It is bactericidal and is an effective chemotherapeutic agent. Its binding has been studied extensively by Nomura, who has shown that it binds to one of the proteins, P_{10}, of the 30s subunit. The presence of streptomycin on the ribosome can cause alterations in the translation process in that "wrong" amino acids are inserted into the growing peptide chain. This is called misreading. It explains the behavior of certain mutants that require either a certain metabolite or streptomycin for growth. In such a mutant, by altering the translation process, streptomycin restores production of a wild-type peptide chain. However, it is unlikely that the killing action of streptomycin is caused by misreading and the subsequent production of "false" proteins. Because of early cessation of protein synthesis after addition of streptomycin and because of the involvement of P_{10} in the initiation process, it is more likely that the killing action of streptomycin is a result of interference with the initiation process.

Streptomycin-resistant mutants of *E. coli* have been isolated in which the P_{10} protein is altered and no longer binds streptomycin. Other mutants in the same gene and affecting the same protein have been found that require streptomycin for growth. In the latter strains, in the absence of streptomycin, mRNA is not read properly, and the presence of streptomycin restores correct reading of mRNA. From these studies it has become clear that the gene altered in streptomycin-resistant and streptomycin-dependent mutants is the structural gene for the ribosomal protein P_{10}. It should be mentioned that by using other antibiotics (for examples, spectinomycin) in a similar way genes for other ribosomal proteins have been located in the immediate vicinity of the gene for P_{10}.

As has been mentioned before (p. 62), streptomycin in whole bacteria inhibits a number of functions. The effects may be consequences secondary to its action on ribosomes. They include damage to the cell membrane, inhibition of RNA and DNA synthesis, and inhibition of respiration. In green plants it causes bleaching presumably because of its selective effect on protein synthesis in chloroplasts.

In addition to puromycin, chloramphenicol, and streptomycin, several other antibiotics are listed in Table 5-3. *Tetracyclines*, which act on the 30s subunit by blocking the binding of aminoacyl-tRNA, are of importance in medicine. *Fusidic acid* inhibits the translocation reaction during peptide-bond elongation. In addition, there are many more antibiotics not listed that act at the level of translation. One of these, *cycloheximide*, inhibits protein synthesis in eukaryotic but not in prokaryotic organisms. Presumably it acts on 80s but not on 70s ribosomes. Its selective action together with that of some of the previously discussed antibiotics is shown in Table 5-4. For further

Table 5-4   Inhibition of Protein Synthesis in Prokaryotes Eukaryotes, and Subcellular Organelles

Antibiotic	Prokaryotes	Eukaryotes	Chloroplasts and/or mitochondria
Chloramphenicol	+	−	+
Streptomycin	+	−	+
Cycloheximide	−	+	−
Puromycin	+	+	+

information on the many antibiotics affecting protein synthesis the reader is referred to articles listed at the end of the chapter. The exact mode of action in the translation process for all of these antibiotics is not known. This reflects as much as anything else on our lack of understanding of the mechanism of protein synthesis.

Antibiotics Affecting Purine Biosynthesis

The pathway of purine biosynthesis is shown in Fig. 5-14. It is very long, leading first to the formation of inosinic acid (IMP), which is a common precursor of guanylic acid (GMP) and adenylic acid (AMP). There are a number of antibiotics that interfere with purine

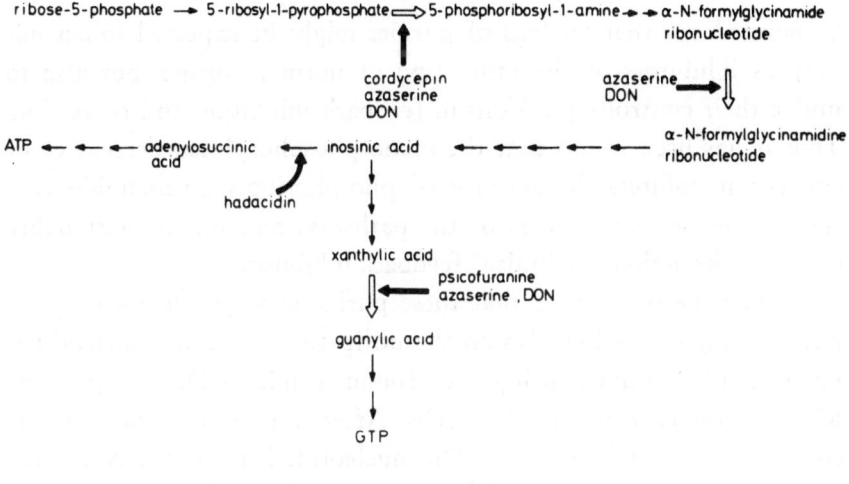

Fig. 5-14. Scheme of purine biosynthesis.

biosynthesis. Their sites of action are indicated in Fig. 5-14 by broad arrows. They fall into two classes: those that act as analogs of precursors of the purine ring (azaserine, 6-diazo-5-oxo-L-norleucine (DON), hadacidin) (Table 3-1), and those that are purine analogs themselves (psicofuranine = angustmycin C, angustmycin A, cordycepin, tubercidin) (Fig. 4-12).

In the first group azaserine and DON are analogs of glutamine, and they interfere with reactions in which glutamine serves as amino donor. For example, they inhibit the steps leading to the formation of 5-phosphoribosylamine and formylglycinamidine ribotide. Hadacidin, an analog of aspartic acid, interferes with the conversion of IMP to adenylosuccinic acid. Curiously, it does not inhibit the formation of 5-amino-4-imidazole-N-succinocarboxamide and is weakly or not at all inhibitory for other cellular reactions involving aspartate.

In the second group psicofuranine and angustmycin A have been shown to inhibit the activity of the enzyme xanthosine-5'-phosphate aminase. The effect is not caused by simple competitive inhibition with the substrate, XMP. Psicofuranine binds to a site on the enzyme different from the active site and causes a conformational change of the enzyme which, though it permits the binding of the normal substrates, prevents the reaction from going to completion. It should be pointed out that analogs of purines might be expected to act not only as inhibitors of the utilization of normal purines, but also to mimic their controlling actions in feedback inhibition and repression. Thus it has been found that the mono-phosphorylated derivative of cordycepin inhibits the activity of phosphoribosylglycinamide synthetase, the second enzyme of the pathway, and this is presumably caused by its action as a "false" feedback inhibitor.

It may be noted here that these purine analogs act not only on purine biosynthesis but also on the utilization of purine nucleotides. For example, cordycepin has been found to inhibit DNA-dependent RNA synthesis in mammalian cells. After uptake, the nucleoside is converted to the triphosphate. This nucleotide is used by RNA polymerase as an analog of ATP. It is incorporated into the growing RNA chain, but since it lacks the 3'-hydroxyl group on the sugar moiety, it cannot act as an acceptor for the next nucleotide. Consequently RNA chain growth is terminated. Cordycepin is therefore listed as an inhibitor of transcription in Table 5-2.

Antibiotics and Iron Metabolism

A number of streptomycetes produce iron-containing antibiotics, called sideromycins. These substances have chemical features in common and form a subgroup of a general class of substances, the siderochromes. In contrast to the sideromycins, siderochromes are produced by many microorganisms. Some of the siderochromes antagonize the effect of sideromycins, and in addition they have a growth-promoting activity on certain microorganisms; these are called sideramines. All the known siderochromes contain iron (Fe^{3+}) linked in a trihydroxamate complex.

Table 3-1 shows an example of a sideromycin, ferrimycin A, and a structurally similar sideramine, ferrioxamine B. Both are aminohydroxylamino-alkane compounds and may be considered as a typical antimetabolite-metabolite pair. Another type of siderochromes, for example, the sideromycin albomycin δ_2, has a polypeptide structure. As far as the sideramines are concerned, the polypeptide type has been obtained only from fungi, whereas the aminohydroxylamino-alkane type has been obtained only from actinomycetes. On the

other hand, both types of sideromycins were obtained from streptomycetes.

Because of the structural similarities between sideromycins and
sideramines and because of the competitive reversal of sideromycin
inhibition by sideramines, it is likely that sideramines are essential
metabolites and that sideromycins inhibit growth by interfering with
their cellular functions. The question arises: What are the reactions in
which sideramines participate? Although the answer has not yet been
found, a few points may help to narrow down the possibilities.

1. The iron-binding capacity seems to be the essential feature of
the function of sideramines: as shown in Table 5-5, sideramines have

Table 5-5 Binding Constants of Various Metal Ion Complexes
of Desterrioxamine B and EDTA

Metal ion	Desferrioxamine	EDTA
	Log K	Log K
Fe^{3+}	30.65	25.1
Ca^{2+}	2.5	10.6
Co^{2+}	10.3	16.1
Zn^{2+}	11.1	16.1
Cu^{2+}	14.2	18.3

a very high affinity for iron, much higher than for other metal ions.
The production of desferri-sideramines by various organisms depends
on the concentration of iron in the medium. It is only under conditions of iron starvation that sideramines are produced in large
amounts. In the presence of iron concentrations that are adequate for
growth, production of sideramines is reduced greatly. Whatever the
role of sideramines turns out to be, it seems highly likely that iron
will be involved in their biochemical function.

2. The chemical structure of the sideramines is such that they can
be excluded as direct participants in electron-transfer systems.

3. On the basis of competitive interactions with sideromycins it
appears that at least one of the sideramine-dependent processes is
essential for growth. Metabolism of resting cells, on the other hand, is
not affected by sideromycins.

Iron is involved in many cellular reactions, and it will be of
interest to see where sideramines will fit into iron metabolism. They

could function either as coenzymes or as iron-carriers that deliver iron to an iron-containing coenzyme or enzyme system. It is probably not until we know the functions of sideramines that we shall understand the mode of action of sideromycins.

References

All Aspects

BÜCHER, TH. and H. SIES, eds., *Inhibitors, Tools in Cell Research*, Springer-Verlag, New York, 1969.

GOTTLIEB, D. and P. D. SHAW, eds., *Antibiotics, I. Mechanism of Action*, Springer-Verlag, New York, 1967.

Granada Symposium on "Mechanism of Action of Antibiotics Against Protein Synthesis and Membranes", edited by Muñoz *et al.* in preparation.

Cell Wall

OSBORN, M. J., "Structure and biosynthesis of the bacterial cell wall," *Ann. Rev. Biochem.* **38**, 501–538, 1969.

GHUYSEN, M. J., "Use of bacteriolytic enzymes in determination of wall structure and their roll in cell metabolism," *Bacterial Rev.* **32**, 425–464, 1968.

Cell Membrane

HAROLD, F. M., *Antimicrobial Agents and Membrane Function. In Advances in Microbial Physiology* **4**, 45–104, Academic Press, Inc., New York, 1970.

Proteins and Nucleic Acids

LEWIN, B. M., *The Molecular Basis of Gene Expression*, Wiley-Interscience, London, 1970.

WATSON, J. D., *Molecular Biology of the Gene*, 2d ed., W. A. BENJAMIN, Inc., New York, 1970.

MAHLER, H. R. and E. H. CORDES, *Biological Chemistry*, Harper and Row, Publishers, New York, 1966.

"The mechanism of protein synthesis," *Cold Spring Harbor Symp. Quant. Biol.* **34**, 1969.

WEISBLUM, B. and J. DAVIES, "Antibiotic inhibitors of the bacterial ribosome," *Bacteriol. Rev.* **32**, 493–528, 1968.

NOMURA, M., "Bacterial ribosome," *Bacteriol. Rev.* **34**, 228–277, 1970.

LEHNINGER, A. L., *Biochemistry. The Molecular Basis of Cell Structure and Function*, Worth Publishers, Inc., New York, 1970.

Siderochromes

SNOW, G. A., "Mycobactins: Iron-chelating growth factors from mycobacteria," *Bacteriol. Rev.* **34**, 99–125, 1970.

KELLER-SCHIERLEIN, W., V. PRELOG and H. ZÄHNER, Siderochrome. *Progress in the Chemistry of Organic Natural Products* **22**, 279, 1964.

Chapter 6

Drug Resistance

General Information

Not all bacterial species are equally sensitive to a given antibiotic. The range of organisms inhibited by an antibiotic is called its antibacterial spectrum. Some antibiotics inhibit growth of a wide variety of organisms ("broad spectrum" antibiotics), whereas others have a narrower antibacterial spectrum, confined to a few groups.

In a population that is sensitive to a given antibiotic, resistant forms can arise through genetic change, either mutation or gene transmission from other cells. Within a species of bacteria we may thus encounter some strains that are sensitive and other strains that are resistant. It has been found that with widespread clinical use of an antibiotic the proportion of resistant strains within a group may rise rapidly. For example, when penicillin was introduced, the proportion of penicillin-resistant staphylococci increased greatly, as shown by the following data, obtained from hospital records:

Year	Percent of total strains that are resistant to penicillin
1946	5
1947/48	17.8
1949	29.1
1950	43.5

After 1950, penicillin was replaced as much as possible by other antibiotics. Subsequently, the fraction of resistant staphylococci decreased:

1951	43
1952	31.3
1953	22.3

It can be surmised from these figures that the emergence of resistant forms in such great proportions may have serious clinical consequences and may limit the usefulness of antibiotics. Many other examples could be cited that illustrate the rapid spread of resistant forms following the introduction of therapy with a given antibiotic. It is especially with R-factor-mediated resistance (see p. 104), which is transmitted by conjugation, that such spreading of resistant strains has been observed during recent years. Here the problem is an especially serious one, because R factors may carry several genes, each of which confers resistance to a different antibiotic. Thus the percent of multiply drug-resistant (streptomycin, tetracycline, chloramphenicol) *Shigellae* isolated in Japan rose from 0.2 in 1954 to 52 in 1964. For these reasons the study of drug resistance has received a great deal of attention. However, the study of drug resistance is also of value for general biological problems, such as the mode of action of antibiotics and the mechanisms of cellular processes in general.

Resistance or sensitivity are not absolute properties of a strain, but are qualities that depend on the concentration of the antibiotic in the medium. As mentioned before (p. 25), for each organism there is a borderline concentration of the antibiotic above which the organism is sensitive and below which it is resistant. Organisms differ from each other in this minimal-inhibitory concentration (MIC). For example, gram-positive bacteria are usually considered to be sensitive to penicillin, whereas gram-negative bacteria are considered resistant. Actually, both are sensitive, but the MIC for most gram-positive bacteria is somewhere near one unit per milliliter, whereas that for most gram-negative bacteria is somewhere near 1000 units per milliliter.

In clinical medicine the consideration of the MIC is of great importance. What is demanded in treatment is the attainment of a concentration of the antibiotic at the site of infection that will inhibit the growth of the pathogen. In determining "sensitivity" or "resistance" of an organism one would like to know if the organism is sufficiently sensitive so that with the available methods of administration, inhibitory concentrations can be reached within the body and especially at the site of infection.

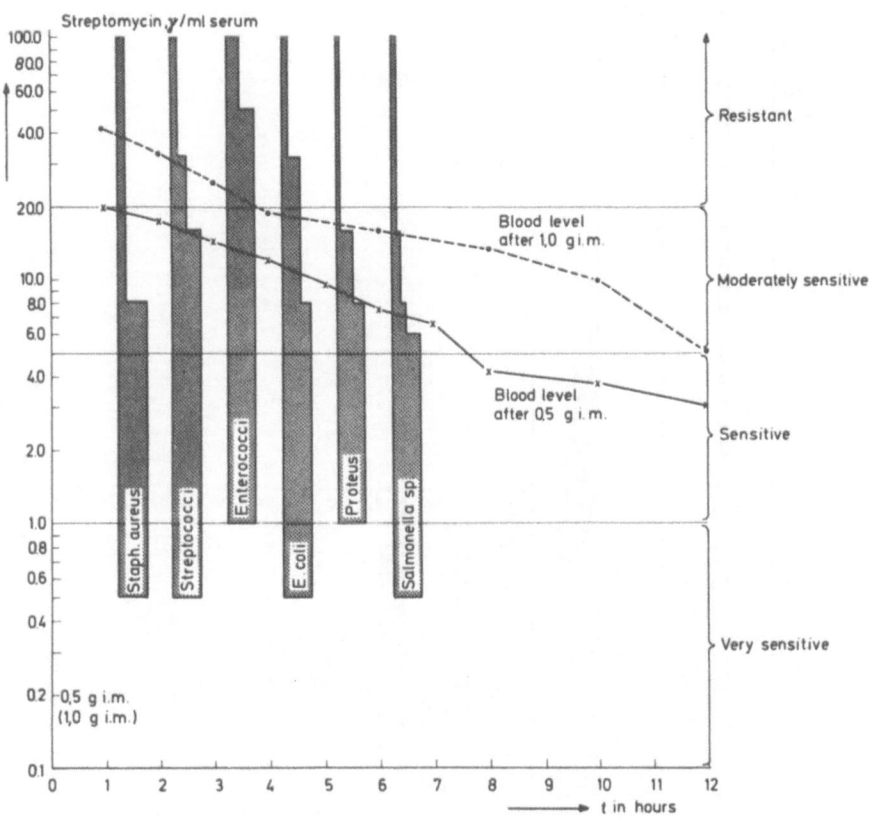

Fig. 6-1. Blood levels of streptomycin after intramuscular administration, and their relationship to the sensitivity of several pathogens. The width of the columns indicates the number of isolates having the indicated sensitivity as determined by serial dilution tests. (From Naumann.)

In Chapter 3 we considered different types of sensitivity tests, and it was pointed out that it is the aim of such tests to give clinically useful information in regard to sensitivity and resistance. Such testing methods aim at finding good correlations between therapeutic effectiveness and the concentration employed in *in vitro* tests. Besides, such methods should be simple and rapid because of the many tests that need to be carried out and because of the importance of starting early treatment. One approach that has been employed to establish the desired correlation is the use of concentrations in the *in vitro* tests that are comparable to the blood levels found after administration of the antibiotic and to classify organisms according to their response to

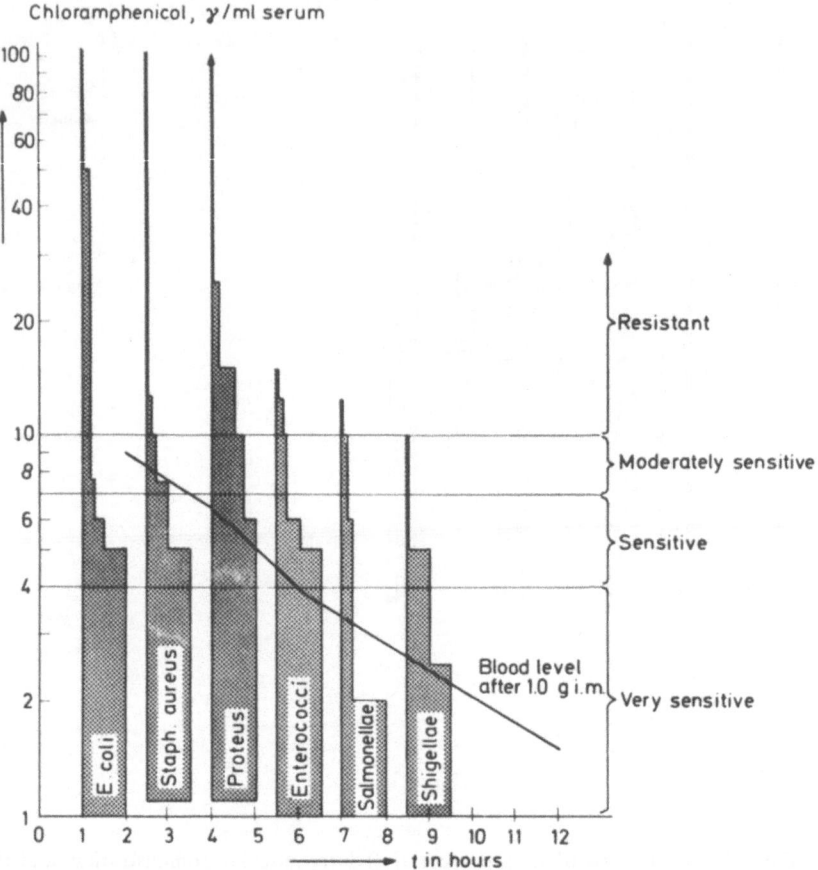

Fig. 6-2. Blood levels of chloramphenicol after intramuscular administration, and their relationship to the sensitivity of several pathogens. See Fig. 6-1. (From Naumann.)

these concentrations of antibiotics. This approach is illustrated in Figs. 6-1 and 6-2 and Tables 6-1 and 6-2 for streptomycin and chloramphenicol. In order to use this approach it is of course necessary to have extensive data on blood levels and also to leave a sufficient margin of safety between the observed MIC and the blood-level concentration to be achieved.

Having made the preceding general comments on drug resistance and its medical implications, we shall now consider the nature of drug-resistant forms in greater detail. Three aspects will be discussed:

Table 6-1 Relationship between Resistance of Pathogen and Therapeutic Dosage of Streptomycin (From Naumann)

Sensitivity of pathogen	Inhibitory concentration range *in vitro*	Dosage required to achieve inhibitory concentration *in vivo*
Very sensitive	Less than 1.0 mg/ml	7 to 10 mg/Kg/day = 0.5 to 0.7 g 250 mg, 2 to 3 times per day
Sensitive	1 to 5 mg/ml	14 to 20 mg/Kg/day = 1 to 1.5 g 500 mg, 2 to 3 times per day
Moderately sensitive	5 to 20 mg/ml	28 to 40 mg/Kg/day = 2 to 3 g 1000 g, 2 to 3 times per day
Resistant	Greater than 20 mg/ml	Impracticable under ordinary conditions; can be achieved topically.

Table 6-2 Relationship between Resistance of Pathogen and Therapeutic Dosage of Chloramphenicol (From Naumann)

Sensitivity of pathogen	Inhibitory concentration range *in vitro*	Dosage required to achieve inhibitory concentration *in vivo*
Very sensitive	Less than 4 mg/ml	20 to 25 mg/Kg/day = about 1.5 g 0.5 g, 3 times per day
Sensitive	4 to 7 mg/ml	30 to 50 mg/Kg/day = about 3 g 1.0 g, 3 times per day
Moderately sensitive	7 to 10 mg/ml	60 to 70 mg/Kg/day = 4 g or more 1.0 to 1.5 g, 4 times per day
Resistant	Greater than 10 mg/ml	Impracticable under ordinary conditions.

(1) the origins of drug-resistant organisms from drug-sensitive ones; (2) the biochemical mechanisms underlying drug resistance; and (3) the control of the emergence and the spread of drug-resistant bacteria.

Origin of Drug-Resistant Forms

Mutation

Mutations to drug resistance have been found for most antibiotics. They occur spontaneously with frequencies of the same order of magnitude as other kinds of mutations, 10^{-6} to 10^{-10} per bacterium. It was shown in the 1940s, mainly through the work of Demerec, that antibiotics do not induce specific mutations conferring resistance but that they act merely as screening agents in suppressing

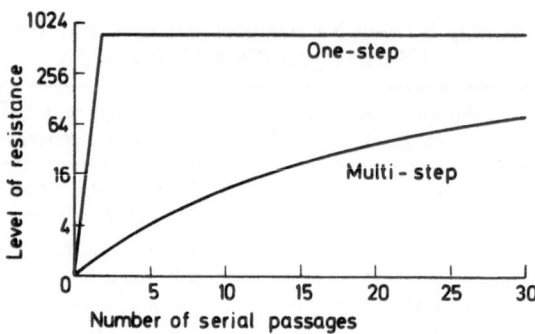

Fig. 6-3. Origin of highly resistant mutants.

the growth of the sensitive cells, thus permitting the outgrowth of resistant mutants present in the population. Such mutant cells had presumably arisen through spontaneous mutation prior to exposure to the antibiotic.

Single mutations can confer either a high degree of resistance or a small increase in resistance. One-step mutants to a high level of resistance have been found with streptomycin, oleandomycin, erythromycin, pikromycin, grisein, ferrimycins, succinimycins, and danomycin. Such mutants may have a 1000-fold greater resistance than their sensitive parents. For most antibiotics, however, such high-level mutations do not occur, and a single mutation increases the level of resistance only moderately (three- to five-fold). In order to build up a high level of resistance for these antibiotics, several mutations have to occur. For example, to build up a 1000-fold increase in resistance to tetracycline, about five consecutive mutations would have to occur. The two modes of origin of resistant mutants are illustrated in Fig. 6-3. For the selection of highly resistant strains, requiring several mutational steps, it is advantageous to grow the bacteria in a chemostat (see p. 18) and to increase the concentration of the antibiotic gradually as populations of an originally low level of resistance are replaced by populations of a higher level of resistance.

In medical practice single-step mutants to a high level of resistance may be troublesome. For example, the emergence of streptomycin-resistant mutants during the treatment of tuberculosis represents a serious problem, especially since treatment is required for a long time. In the case of mutations to low levels of resistance, on the other hand, outgrowth of resistant mutants can be prevented by maintaining an adequate blood level — higher than that to which a single-step mutant would be resistant. (The chance for two mutations to occur in the same cell is extremely small.) It is also important, especially with bacteristatic antibiotics, to prevent a lowering of the blood level during therapy.

Genetic Transfer

In bacteria, three types of genetic transfer mechanisms have been found: transformation, involving transfer of "naked" DNA; transduction, in which the DNA from the donor is carried to the recipient inside a phage; and conjugation, which requires contact of donor and recepient cells and in which the genetic material is transferred through a channel between the two mating cells. For the transfer of drug-resistance genes only transduction and conjugation are of importance. Transduction is the mechanism of transfer in staphylococci. Conjugation is involved in transfer of resistance genes among various groups of *Enterobacteriaceae.*

In both types of organisms the genes for drug resistance are carried not only on the chromosome but also on extrachromosomal elements or plasmids. These are about 1 to 2 percent the size of the chromosome, and like the chromosome, they are circular. They are independent "replicons" — they have a genetic system that controls their own replication. Many of the plasmids of enteric bacteria, which, as we have mentioned, are called R factors, also contain genes that are involved in the promotion of their own transfer to recipient cells. These R factors, therefore, belong to the general category of sex factors, of which the F factor of *E.'coli* is the best-studied example.

Plasmid-carried resistance genes for several commonly used antibiotics have been found in pathogenic staphylococci. These include genes conferring resistance to penicillin, erythromycin, chloramphenicol, tetracycline, and kanamycin. Some are linked together on the same plasmid (penicillin and erythromycin); others are on separate plasmids. Staphylococci carrying such plasmids are usually lysogenic for temperate phages, which can act as transducing vectors for the transfer of the plasmids. That transduction may be responsible for the acquisition of drug resistance in disease was demonstrated in mice infected with genetically marked resistant and sensitive strains. It was possible to isolate from kidneys of the mice, bacteria that had received plasmids carrying the genes for penicillin and erythromycin resistance.

R factors have been studied extensively during the last decade. Here again, genes conferring resistance to a variety of commonly used antibiotics and other chemotherapeutic agents are found: chloramphenicol, tetracycline, streptomycin, penicillin, kanamycin, neomycin, polymyxin, and sulfonamides. These genes are found in a variety of combinations on different R factors, a given R factor carrying one or several resistance genes. In addition to carrying different combinations of such genes, R factors have also been found to differ from each other in the genes controlling functions necessary for genetic transfer. R factors can be transmitted not only to members of the same species but also to cells of other related species. Thus the group of organisms that can act as hosts for R factors includes *Shigella, Salmonella, Proteus, E. coli, Aerobacter, Serratia,* and *V. cholerae.* Thus R factors can be transmitted from a pathogenic organism, such as *Shigella,* to a nonpathogen, such as *E. coli,* and back again to other pathogens. This type of transfer has been demonstrated in experiments with germ-free mice. *E. coli,* a common inhabitant of the human bowel, can act as a reservoir of R factors and render infecting enteric pathogens resistant. R factors have spread recently not only within Japan, but also throughout the rest of the world, including Europe and America, and a large fraction of enteric pathogens isolated during recent years carry R factors. One circumstance that has contributed to the spread of R factors is the use of antibiotics in animal feeds. This practice selects for the outgrowth of resistant organisms in farm animals, and such strains may be transferred to humans through the eating of raw meats or meat products. In Great Britain, legislation has recently been passed that prohibits the use of the major chemotherapeutic agents in animal feeds. This legislation was based on a careful study by a committee of biologists appointed by the government to investigate possible hazards arising from the use of antibiotics in animal feeds and veterinary medicine. The report of the committee has been published (see references).

Some R factors can become dissociated into a nontransmissible portion, carrying the resistance genes and a transmissible portion, called RTF, carrying the sex factor genes but lacking resistance genes. These two entities can replicate independently in a cell. The RTF element may be transferred to other cells without the resistance determinants. However, the two elements may also become associated during transfer and may be transmitted together.

Biochemical Mechanisms of Drug Resistance

In order to discuss the ways in which a bacterium may become resistant to the action of an antibiotic, we use the following diagram.

$$S \xrightarrow[A]{E} P$$

The substrate, S, is converted to the product, P. The reaction is catalyzed by the enzyme, E, and the activity of E is inhibited by the antibiotic, A. Mutation to resistance may involve the following types of changes:

1. a change in E so that it is no longer inhibited by A;

2. increased production of S in cases where A and S compete for a site on E;

3. a reaction at another site that prevents A from reaching E, (this includes destruction or inactivation of A);

4. a change in metabolism so that P is no longer essential for growth.

An example of an altered target site of an antibiotic is the mutation to streptomycin resistance affecting the protein P10 of the 30s ribosomal subunit (p. 91). Although no enzymatic function has been demonstrated for P10, it has been shown to be required for initiation of translation. In streptomycin-sensitive strains streptomycin binds to this protein. In streptomycin-resistant strains it no longer binds to P10. Yet the altered P10 is still able to function in protein synthesis. As mentioned previously, another mutation involving the same gene results in a requirement of streptomycin for growth. In such streptomycin-dependent mutants, the P10 protein is also altered, but it still binds streptomycin. Presumably the alteration is such that streptomycin bound to the P10 protein is essential for the initiation of translation.

Another example of an altered target site as a result of a mutation to resistance, in this case an enzyme, is provided by a class of cana-

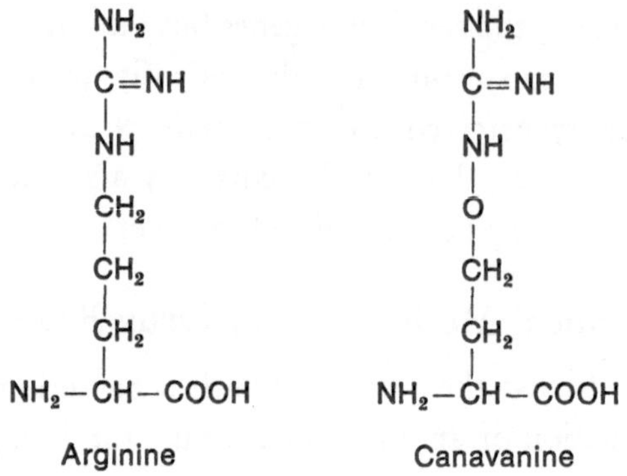

```
        NH₂                      NH₂
         |                        |
        C=NH                     C=NH
         |                        |
        NH                       NH
         |                        |
        CH₂                       O
         |                        |
        CH₂                      CH₂
         |                        |
        CH₂                      CH₂
         |                        |
NH₂—CH—COOH              NH₂—CH—COOH

     Arginine                 Canavanine
```

Fig. 6-4. Structure of arginine and canavanine.

vanine-resistant mutants of *E. coli*. Canavanine, a product of jack beans, is a structural analog of arginine (Fig. 6-4) and inhibits growth by competing with arginine for the arginine-activating enzyme (arginyl-tRNA synthetase). Resistant mutants possessing an activating enzyme with reduced affinity for arginine and canavanine have been isolated. In such mutants the ability to synthesize arginyl-tRNA is reduced, but it is still sufficient to permit growth, especially with added arginine.

The same system can also provide an example of the second type of mechanism mentioned above, increased production of S. Among canavanine-resistant mutants isolated, strains have been found that overproduce arginine and excrete it into the culture medium. The strains harbor mutations in a regulator gene that controls repressibility of the enzymes of arginine biosynthesis. In such mutants, arginine is no longer able to repress the formation of the arginine-biosynthetic enzymes, with the result that arginine production is greatly increased.

The third type of mechanism of drug-resistance includes several types of changes: altered permeability, chemical modification of the antibiotic, and destruction of the antibiotic. Most of the plasmid-mediated resistances fall into this category.

For clinically important antibiotics, permeability changes as a result of mutation have been claimed, but thorough experimental documentation is lacking. For example, in certain tetracycline-resistant and chloramphenicol-resistant mutants resistance has been as-

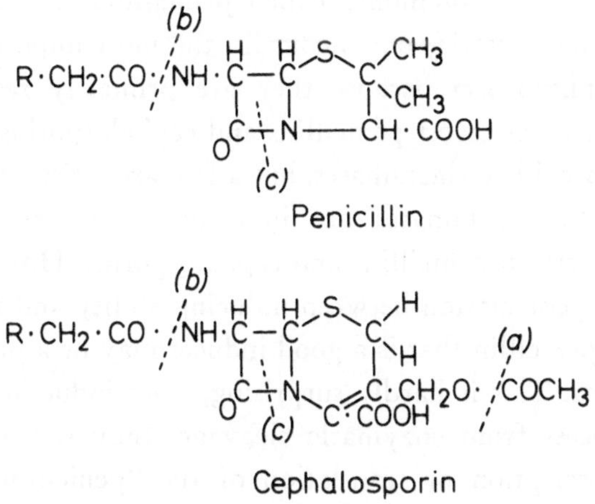

Penicillin

Cephalosporin

Fig. 6-5. Action of enzymes attacking penicillins and cephalosporins. (a) Acyl-esterases; (b) amidases; (c) β-lactamases. (From Citri, N. and M. R. Pollock, "The biochemistry and function of β-lactamase (penicillinase)," *Advan. Enzymol.* **28,** 237—321, 1966.

cribed to reduced transport of the antibiotic into the cell. Here again the canavanine-arginine system supplies a well-documented example. A class of canavanine-resistant mutants was found to be deficient in the transport of the basic amino acids, arginine, ornithine, lysine and presumably canavanine into the cell. For arginine, ornithine, and lysine the defect could be observed by reduced rate of uptake of radioactive amino acids into the soluble pool of the cells. It may be noted in passing that the example of the different classes of canava-nine-resistant mutants show how each of several completely unrelated alterations in metabolism, involving different genes, can lead to the same end result: resistance to the growth-inhibitory action of an antibiotic.

There are a number of systems in which the mechanism of drug resistance involves destruction of the antibiotic. Of these the one best studied is penicillin resistance. There are two groups of enzymes that degrade penicillins and cephalosporins, beta-lactamases and amidases. In addition there are acyl esterases that split cephalosporins. The bonds cleaved as a result of the action of these enzymes are indicated in Fig. 6-5.

Beta-lactamases, commonly called penicillinases, are widely distributed among bacteria, but medically the most important ones are those of staphylococci because they are primarily responsible for penicillin resistance. Most penicillins and cephalosporins are sensitive to staphylococcal beta-lactamases, but a few are resistant (methicillin, cloxacillin). Beta-lactamases are inducible enzymes, the inducing agents being certain penicillins and cephalosporins. However, there is no one-to-one correlation between inducing ability and function as a substrate. A penicillin that is a good inducer may be a poor substrate, and vice versa. This is hardly surprising, since induction is a totally different process from enzymatic cleavage. Induction occurs at the level of transcription or translation of the "penicillinase operon," whereas cleavage occurs after the finished protein molecule has been released from the ribosomes.

The genes for beta-lactamase production in staphylococci may be carried on a plasmid or on the chromosome. Extensive studies have been carried out on the genetics of the plasmid-controlled beta-lactamase. This genetic system contains both structural and regulatory genes, closely linked to each other. In gram-negative bacteria, such as *E. coli*, beta-lactamase production has also been found to be controlled by either chromosomal or plasmid (R-factor) genes. These findings of either a chromosomal or a plasmid location have suggested the possibility that resistance genes carried by plasmids may originally have had a chromosomal location and may have acquired a plasmid location secondarily.

The other enzymes that split penicillins and cephalosporins are also widely distributed among microorganisms, but neither the amidases nor the acyl esterases seem to play a clinically important role in drug resistance. The amidases are of practical importance because they liberate the 6-amino-penicillanic "nucleus" from penicillins by removing the natural side chain; they thus furnish an important starting substance for the preparation of semisynthetic penicillins.

For a number of antibiotics a mechanism of resistance has been found that involves coupling of the drug with another compound to form an inactive derivative. In most of these cases the genes for the production of such "detoxifying" enzymes are carried on R factors.

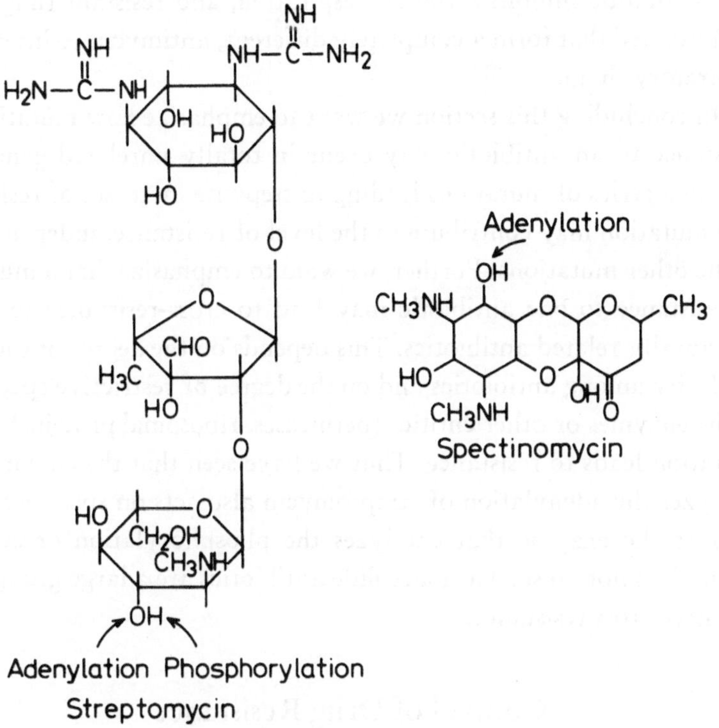

Fig. 6-6. Structures of streptomycin and spectinomycin. Sites of adenylation and phosphorylation are indicated.

Thus R-factor mediated resistance to chloramphenicol involves production of an acetylating enzyme which, with acetyl CoA as acetyl donor, catalyzes the production of mono- and diacetyl derivatives of chloramphenicol. For streptomycin two such enzymes have been described, one which leads to the adenylation of streptomycin and also of spectinomycin, the other which leads to the phosphorylation of streptomycin, without affecting spectinomycin or other aminoglycoside antibiotics (see Fig. 6-6).

The last general mechanism of drug resistance, creation of a metabolic shunt that bypasses the inhibited reaction, has often been claimed, especially in the early days of antibiotics, but there are very few documented cases of this mechanism and it does not seem to be of medical importance. One case is resistance to antimycin A in fungi.

This antibiotic inhibits terminal respiration, and resistant fungi have been isolated that form a completely different, antimycin A-insensitive respiratory chain.

In concluding this section we want to emphasize how mutations to resistance to an antibiotic may occur in totally unrelated genes and how in a series of mutations leading to stepwise increases of resistance each mutation may contribute to the level of resistance, independently of the other mutations. Further, we want to emphasize that a mutation to resistance to one antibiotic may lead to cross-resistance to other, structurally related antibiotics. This depends on the degree of chemical similarity among antibiotics and on the degree of restrictive specificity of the enzymes or other entities (permeases, ribosomal proteins) whose alteration leads to resistance. Thus we have seen that the enzyme that catalyzes the adenylation of streptomycin also acts on spectinomycin, whereas the enzyme that catalyzes the phosphorylation of streptomycin does not do so. The macrolide antibiotics are a large group with extensive cross resistance.

Control of Drug Resistance

We shall consider the problem of combating drug resistance under three subheadings: (1) prevention of the emergence of drug-resistant forms during therapy; (2) prevention of the spreading of resistant forms; and (3) elimination of resistant forms after they have emerged during treatment. The emphasis will be on the first two aspects, as the last aspect may be considered as a "rear-guard" action rather than an attack on the problem.

Prevention of the Emergence of Drug-Resistant Organisms

We have already mentioned the danger of the outgrowth of drug-resistant mutants during the prolonged treatment of tuberculosis with streptomycin. To combat this one can use combined therapy with two or more unrelated drugs. For example, combinations of streptomycin with p-amino-salicylic acid (PAS) or with isoniazid may be used. Assuming that the frequency of a mutation to resistance for each drug alone is 10^{-6} per bacterium, the expected frequency of a double mutation to resistance against both drugs is 10^{-12} per bacterium. In view of the numbers of bacteria involved in an infection the chance for a double mutant to arise is very small. In practice, it is of course essential that both drugs are present at inhibitory levels at the site of infection.

Prevention of the Spreading of Resistant Forms

Within a given environment the more an antibiotic is used, the greater the chance that populations of resistant bacteria will replace populations of sensitive ones. For example, in hospitals, where antibiotics are used widely, it has been found that a large fraction of enteric strains carried by hospital personnel are resistant to various antibiotics. This increases the probability of superinfection of patients with resistant organisms. We have mentioned before that the use of antibiotics in animal feeds has led to a great increase in drug-resistant strains of animal origin. The problem ist aggravated by the rapid spread of multiple drug resistance made possible by transmissible resistance factors.

In order to fight against the spread of drug-resistant forms it is necessary to limit the use of antibiotics as much as possible. We have mentioned that in the case of farm animals, only those antibiotics should be used that are not used in clinical medicine. In the case of hospitals, rotation in the use of antibiotics has been employed. As was shown before, (p. 97), when use of an antibiotic is discontinued, the frequency of resistant strains decreases. For example, one may put antibiotics into three groups:

Group I	Group II	Group III
Tetracyclines	Penicillin	Vancomycin
Macrolides	Streptomycin	Ristocetin
Sulfonamides	Chloramphenicol	Neomycin
		Colistin
		Polymyxin
		Kanamycin

Groups I and II may be used alternately in three-to-four year cycles, whereas the antibiotics in Group III are kept in reserve for special cases. However, because of the recent increase in travel, the migration of people in industrialized countries, and the concomitant spread of resistant organisms, this type of approach has lost some of its effectiveness.

Elimination of Resistant Forms during Treatment

If in the course of antibiotic therapy resistant forms grow out, it becomes necessary to switch to another drug to which the infectious agent is sensitive. For example, if resistance to penicillin develops because of the emergence of a penicillinase-producing strain, one can switch to a penicillinase-resistant penicillin, such as methicillin or cloxacillin. However, such switching may be hazardous because when treatment is urgently required there may not be enough time to carry out sensitivity tests. The situation is aggravated by the possibility that the resistant strain may carry a plasmid with several resistance genes.

As we mentioned before, resistance may develop against most of the antibiotics so that the search for new antibiotics, for which there are no resistant forms, is most likely only a temporary stop gap. Besides, with more and more antibiotics becoming available, it becomes almost impossible for physicians to have detailed knowledge of all of the agents at their disposal. A further complication is the marketing of preparations containing combinations of antibiotics, with each such combination having its individual trade name.

Microbial Persistence

Before concluding this chapter, the phenomenon of "microbial persistence" should be mentioned. It has been defined by McDermott as "the capacity of microbes to survive drug exposure in the tissues despite susceptibility to the drug *in vitro*." In other words, some pathogens in the body are not affected by the antibiotic, either because they are protected by their surroundings or because they are at a stage of their life cycle at which they are refractory to the inhibition by the antibiotic. For example, they may be located in an area, such as the inside of a cell, to which the antibiotic cannot penetrate. Or they may be in the stationary phase of growth so that they are not affected by those antibiotics that require growth of the organisms to be effective.

Thus some organisms may exist temporarily in a spheroplast or L-form state and may be protected against cell-wall antibiotics, such as penicillins.

Persistence of pathogens can be responsible for relapse if therapy is discontinued too early. It is thus necessary to take the possibility of persistence into account when prescribing a course of therapy. Like drug resistance, persistence entails the survival of pathogens during treatment. The two phenomena are, however, basically different; drug resistance involves the survival and outgrowth of a genetically different population. Persistence involves escape from the drug action of some sensitive individuals within a genetically homogeneous population. If for one reason or another these individuals leave their "protected state," they will be subject to the drug's inhibitory action.

References

CITRI, N. and M. R. POLLOCK, "The biochemistry and function of β-lactamase (penicillinase), *Advan. Enzymol.* **28**, 237–321, 1966.

DULANEY, E. L. and A. I. LASKIN, eds., *The Problems of Drug-Resistant Pathogenic Bacteria*. Annals of the New York Academy of Sciences. **182**, 1971.

MITSUHASHI, S., *Transferable Drug Resistance Factor R*, University Park Press, Baltimore, 1971.

NAUMANN, P., "Antibiotica, Blutspiegel and Resistenzbestimmung," *Antibiotica et Chemotherapia*, Fortschr. **10**, 1—93, 1962.

WOLSTENHOLME, G. E. W. and M. O'CONNOR, eds., *Bacterial Episomes and Plasmids*, J. and A. Churchill Ltd., London, 1969.

Joint Committee on the Use of Antibiotics in Animal Husbandry and Veterinary Medicine, Report Command No. 4190, Her Majesty's Stationary Office, London, 1969 (The "Swann Report").

Chapter 7

The Future of Antibiotics

Is the Search for New Antibiotics Justified?

Assuming that the search for new antibiotics continues, at some future time all the useful antibiotics will have been found. In the screening procedures employed for new antibiotics one of the major tasks has become the sorting out of "rediscovered" compounds from new ones, and this task is becoming increasingly difficult as more antibiotics become known. Have we already reached the point where the yield of useful new antibiotics is not worth the effort of obtaining them? In trying to evaluate this question we can list a number of arguments in favor of continuing the search for new antibiotics at the present time.

1. So far the search for antibiotics has been largely empirical, involving the screening of strains isolated from nature for antibacterial activity. Most antibiotics are products of secondary metabolism, and this type of metabolism, like primary metabolism, is under genetic control. There are thus unlimited possibilities for the isolation of mutants, not only with increased antibiotic production but with altered pathways leading to the formation of new products. As our knowledge of these pathways increases, it becomes possible to look for mutants in more rational and meaningful ways. This applies especially to mutations affecting control mechanisms, such as enzyme-repression and feedback-inhibition. For example, with mutants derepressed for a primary pathway of biosynthesis one may find new secondary pathways opening up as a result of the overproduction of intermediates along the primary pathway.

Genetic crosses will be valuable in obtaining desirable combinations of mutations. Mating procedures are well worked-out with those fungi in which the sexual stage of the life cycle is known. However, this applies to only a few of the antibiotic-producing species. For bacteria as a whole, the elucidation of mating systems is still at a rudimentary stage, and in only a few species has genetic analysis been developed extensively. Among actinomycetes, genetic analysis by crosses can be carried out in *Streptomyces coelicolor* and *S. rimosus* and a linkage map is available for these organisms. Among *Bacilli*, genetic analysis by transformation and transduction can be carried out in *B. subtilis*, but little is known about genetic systems of the major antibiotic-producing *Bacilli*. In summary, for the secondary metabolism of antibiotic-producing organisms, biochemical genetics with the degree of sophistication achieved in work on primary metabolism is largely a task for the future.

2. The success of antibiotics has been mainly in the area of bacterial and, to some extent, fungal infections. There are many other diseases for which no or not very effective antibiotics have been found. These include viral, protozoal, and helminthic infections, and neoplastic disease. Many antibiotics have been described for the last category, but none is comparable in its effectiveness to the major antibacterial antibiotics. With most of these diseases, selective toxicity is much more difficult to achieve than with bacterial or fungal infections.

3. Even in the case of bacterial infections there are a number of problems that demand the isolation of new antibiotics. First, the increased incidence of resistant strains makes it necessary to find other antibiotics to which bacteria are still sensitive. Second, some antibiotics produce undesirable effects, which might be avoided by substituting new antibiotics. For example, broad-spectrum antibiotics eliminate not only pathogens but also the normal flora of the body, and this makes the host susceptible to superinfection by other microbes, such as *Candida*, a yeast, which is not sensitive to these antibiotics. Such difficulties might be avoided by using antibiotics that have either an even broader spectrum that includes yeasts or have a narrower, more specific spectrum for the pathogen in question, without affecting the members of the normal flora.

4. Antibiotics find increasing use in areas besides medicine, such as animal nutrition, preservation of foods, protection of plants (fungicides and insecticides), and laboratory investigations. As we have mentioned, the widespread use of an antibiotic fosters the emergence

of resistant strains. It thus becomes important to look for antibiotics that are different from the ones used in clinical medicine and for which there is no cross-resistance with chemotherapeutic agents and no genetically transmissible resistance.

5. Antibiotics have gained increasing usefulness as tools in biochemical investigations. Like mutations, they produce specific lesions in metabolism and can thus be used as "intracellular dissecting needles" to work out the steps of metabolic pathways. As we shall discuss presently, the search for antibiotics useful for these purposes demands somewhat different selection procedures than are employed for the isolation of therapeutic agents; such procedures may unearth new classes of naturally occurring compounds.

Methods Used in the Search for New Antibiotics

We shall consider two approaches here: (1) screening procedures for antibiotics produced by wild-type strains or mutants, and (2) modification of already existing antibiotics.

Screening of Strains for the Production of New Antibiotics

Before considering the methods used for screening, we shall comment briefly on the choice of organisms to be tested as sources of antibiotics. As most antibiotics are secondary metabolites, the more we know about the secondary metabolism of an organism, the better we are qualified to evaluate the chance of finding new antibiotics. This applies especially to our ability to predict the properties of mutants that might be isolated. On a more empirical level, it might be expected that organisms that produce a variety of antibiotics have a greater potential for producing yet unknown ones than organisms that produce only one or a few antibiotics. The greatest variety of antibiotics is found among actinomycetes and *Aspergillales,* and these groups may therefore be considered favorable starting material for new antibiotics. A possible disadvantage is that so many of their antibiotics are already known, but the extension of screening for antibiotics to mutant strains might outweigh the advantages of using a less-well-known organism with a presumably lower genetic potential for the production of antibiotics.

In the selection of naturally occurring strains as sources of antibiotics the source of the inoculum (usually soil) for isolation may affect the variety of organisms obtained. As a general rule, the diversity of plant life correlates well with the diversity of the microbial flora. Thus cultivated soils in temperate climates usually contain a large number of microbes but a relatively small variety, whereas soils from tropical climates usually contain a smaller number but a greater variety.

The next problem, after the choice of strains has been made, is the selection of testing methods and, closely connected with that, selection of methods for classifying and identifying potentially new antibiotics. Ideally, one would like testing methods to have the following properties: (1) rapid, reproducible execution, involving a minimun amount of labor; (2) sensitivity toward many antibiotics; (3) ability to recognize new antibiotics without interference from antibiotics already known; and (4) correlation between the test result and the effectiveness in the treatment of disease.

In regard to the first property, simple and effective methods are available for the detection of antibiotics. As an example, in Chapter 3 we have described the cross-streak test. With a slight modification, the plate-diffusion test illustrated in Fig. 7-1 can also be used. Here, the sources of the antibiotics are cultures of actinomycetes, and the test organism is *B. subtilis.*

In regard to sensitivity toward many antibiotics, this depends on the choice of the testing organisms and the nature of the culture medium. In general, microorganisms are more susceptible in chemically defined "minimal" media than in complex "rich" media. This is because the action of many antibiotics is reversed by metabolites present in rich media. For example, 40 to 60 percent of actinomycetes isolated show an antibiotic activity against *B. subtilis* in a rich medium. By using minimal media and a variety of test organisms, including gram-negative bacteria and fungi, one can demonstrate at least one and sometimes several antibiotic activities for every actinomycete tested. When such a plethora of antibiotics is produced, it is desirable to have rapid and efficient methods for identification, especially methods that do not require prior concentration of the antibiotic (see below).

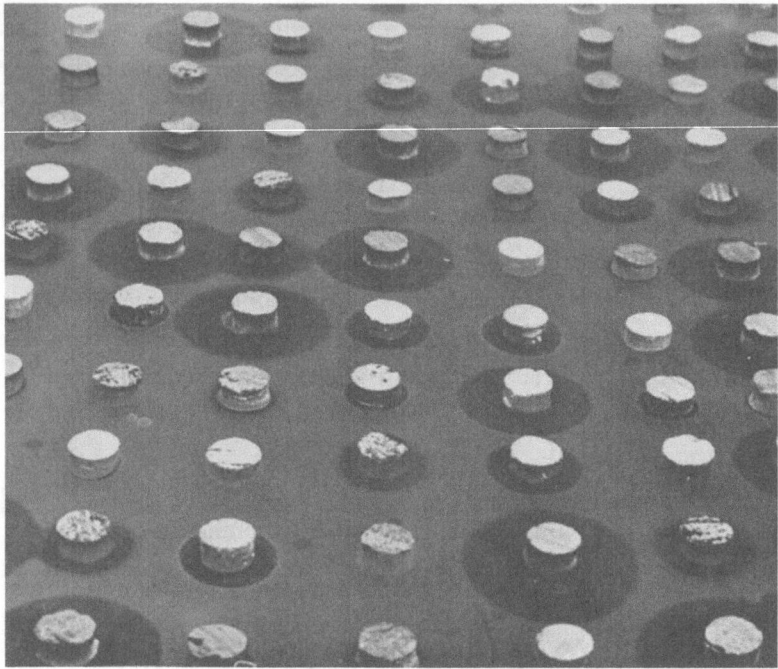

Fig. 7-1. Plate-diffusion test for the detection of new antibiotics. Agar blocks containing mycelium of actinomycetes to be screened are placed on an agar medium seeded with *B. subtilis.*

To differentiate between new and already-known antibiotics is a difficult problem, in view of the large number of antibiotics already described. One way to avoid rediscovery of at least the common antibiotics is to use resistant strains as test organisms. Of particular value in this regard are strains carrying a plasmid that contains genes specifying resistance for several unrelated antibiotics.

Finally, to detect new antibiotics that have a good chance of being effective against human infections it is helpful to use human pathogens as indicator strains. This applies especially to situations in which one is looking for an antibiotic against a specific pathogen. For example, in order to find an agent effective against the disease favus, it is advisable to employ the causative agent, *Trichophyton*, as a test organism. This organism is difficult to grow. If one is interested in obtaining a general antifungal agent, it may be more advantageous to use a fungus as an indicator strain that is easier to grow, even though this fungus may not be as specific an indicator strain for chemotherapeutically valuable antibiotics. In passing, it should be noted that there are a number of pathogens that cannot be grown *in vitro* (plasmodia, rickettsiae), and they are therefore unsuitable as indicator strains.

As more and more antibiotics become known, simple methods for rapid identification are becoming increasingly crucial in distinguishing old antibiotics from new ones. At the present time 40 to 50 new antibiotics are described every year, and the total number of antibiotics that have been characterized is well over a thousand. The main difficulties encountered in the rapid identification of an antibiotic are (a) interference from impurities in the culture filtrate; (b) the possibility that several different antibiotics are present in such a filtrate; and (c) insufficiently accurate and relevant information about known antibiotics, for purposes of comparison with the presumptive new antibiotic. However, a number of useful procedures help to establish the identity of an antibiotic, and these are based largely on comparisons with the properties of known antibiotics.

Identification of an antibiotic involves two general stages: (1) assignment to a general group and (2) comparison with other members of the group to which it has been assigned in order to see whether or not it is identical with a known compound.

The attainment of stage one can usually be achieved by determining a number of biological properties of the antibiotic. Purification is not required for this purpose. The properties include its antibacterial spectrum, cross-resistance with other antibiotics, and reversal of its inhibitor action by known substances. Other considerations of its biological origin help to narrow down the number of possible groups, according to the "rule of specificity," discussed in Chapter 2.

Once an antibiotic has been assigned to a group, one must purify it before he attempts to achieve stage 2. Conventional techniques of analytical chemistry can be used to compare it with other antibiotics. These include various kinds of chromatography and electrophoresis. We should recall here the technique of bioautography (see p. 65), which consists of paper chromatography, thin-layer chromatography, or paper electrophoresis, combined with growth response of susceptible organisms, and which, because of its specificity, is especially useful for identification of biologically active substances. Final identification can be achieved only with a pure preparation and should be based on the usual chemical and physical criteria, such as NMR spectroscopy, mass spectroscopy, UV and infrared spectra. Careful characterization of the pure compound is especially important for substances in which identity with a known antibiotic has not been established, for it is this information that permanently establishes the compound as a new antibiotic and thus serves as a guide for future work.

Modification of Already-Existing Antibiotics

The approach of obtaining improved "new" antibiotics by the modification of already-existing ones has had variable success. For some antibiotics it has worked very well; for others is has been a failure. For example, chloramphenicol is easily synthesized, and hundreds of derivatives and similar compounds have been prepared. Yet none of these is a marked improvement over chloramphenicol itself in regard to either antibacterial or to pharmacological properties. On the other hand, many useful derivatives of 6-aminopenicillanic acid have been prepared. This compound can be isolated either as a fermentation product or by enzymatic cleavage of penicillins. Some of the semisynthetic penicillins derived from 6-aminopenicillanic acid are listed in Table 7-1, together with some of the naturally occurring penicillins. The table shows the properties that make them more desirable than naturally occurring penicillins.

In concluding this chapter we may note that of the many antibiotics discovered in the past, only a small fraction — not more than 5 percent — are of therapeutic value. Hopefully, as our knowledge of metabolism increases, more rational selection procedures will result in a higher proportion of therapeutically useful substances. In addition, antibiotics fulfill other functions besides serving as therapeutic agents. As we have pointed out, they are valuable tools for prying into processes occurring in living cells. Beyond that, their mere existence poses interesting questions in regard to metabolism, and possibly ecology. It is our hope that this little volume will have roused the interest of the reader in these substances and will make him wonder about the reasons for the existence of antibiotics.

Table 7-1   Therapeutically Important Properties of Penicillins

$$R-N(H)-CH-CH \diagup S \diagdown C(CH_3)(CH_3)$$
$$C-N-CHCOOH$$
$$\| O$$

	Effective Against				
	Gram-positive bacteria	Gram-negative bacteria	Penicillinase producing staph	Orally effective (acid-resistant)	Induction of penicillinase
Natural					
Penicillin G	++	−	−	−	+
$R = \langle \rangle -CH_2C(=O)-$					
Penicillin V	++	−	−	+	+
$R = \langle \rangle -O-CH_2C(=O)-$					
Semisynthetic					
Methicillin	+	−	+	−	++
$R = \langle \rangle (OCH_2)(OCH_3) -C(=O)-$					
Oxacillin	++	−	++	+	+++
$R = \langle \rangle -C(=N)-C-C(=O)-$, $C-CH_3$, O					
Ampicillin	++	+	−	+	+
$R = \langle \rangle -CH(NH_2)-C(=O)-$					

References

Therapeutically Useful Antibiotics

EVANS, R. M., *The Chemistry of Antibiotics Used in Medicine*, Pergamon Press, Inc., London, 1965.

GARROD, L. P. and F. O'GRADY, *Antibiotic and Chemotherapy*, E. and S. Livingstone, Ltd., Edinburgh, 1968.

SCHNITZER, R. J. and F. HAWKING, eds., *Experimental Chemotherapy*, Academic Press, Inc., New York, 1964.

WALTER, A. M. and L. HEILMEYER, *Antibiotica–Fibel*. 3d ed., Thieme Verlag, Stuttgart, 1968.

Search for New Antibiotics

HEROLD, M. and Z. GABRIEL, eds., *Antibiotics. Advances in Research, Production and Clinical Use*, Butterworth & Co. (Publishers) Ltd., London, 1966.

SEVCIK, V., *Antibiotica aus Actinomyceten*, G. Fischer Verlag, Jena, 1963.

WAKSMAN, S. A., "Success and failures in the search for antibiotics," *Advan. Appl. Microbiol.* 11, 1–16, 1969. See other papers on antibiotics in the same volume.

Progress in Antimicrobial and Anticancer Chemotherapy, Proceedings of the 6th International Congress of Chemotherapy, Tokyo, 2 vols., University Park Press, Baltimore, 1970.

Periodicals

	Most recent volume
Antibiotiki, Eksperim. Klinich. Izuch. Sb. Rabot	15, 1970
Hindustan Antibiot. Bull.	12 and 13, 1970
J. Antibiotics (Tokoyo). Series A in English, Series B in Japanese	23, 1970
Antimicrobial Agents Ann.	10, 1970

Index

(Italic numbers refer to figures or tables)

123